Dawning Answers

DAWNING ANSWERS

How the HIV/AIDS Epidemic Has Helped to Strengthen Public Health

Edited by

Ronald O. Valdiserri, M.D., M.P.H.

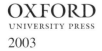

OXFORD
UNIVERSITY PRESS

2003

OXFORD
UNIVERSITY PRESS

Oxford   New York
Auckland   Bangkok   Buenos Aires   Cape Town   Chennai
Dar es Salaam   Delhi   Hong Kong   Istanbul   Karachi   Kolkata
Kuala Lumpur   Madrid   Melbourne   Mexico City   Mumbai
Nairobi   São Paulo   Shanghai   Taipei   Tokyo   Toronto

Copyright © 2003 by Oxford University Press, Inc.

Published by Oxford University Press, Inc.
198 Madison Avenue, New York, New York, 10016
http://www.oup-usa.org

Oxford is a registered trademark of Oxford University Press

Library of Congress Cataloging-in-Publication Data
Dawning answers : how the HIV/AIDS epidemic has helped
to strengthen public health /
edited by Ronald O. Valdiserri.
p. cm.   Includes bibliographical references and index.
ISBN 0-19-514740-5 (cloth)
1. AIDS (Disease). 2. Public health.
I. Valdiserri, Ronald O., 1951–
RA643.8.D395 2003   362.1'969792—dc21   2002025033

9 8 7 6 5 4 3 2 1

Printed in the United States of America
on acid-free paper

For Edwina and Ronald,

La riconoscenza e la memoria del cuore

Preface

So many superlatives have been used to describe human immunodeficiency virus (HIV) infection and the acquired immunodeficiency syndrome (AIDS): the greatest epidemic of modern times; an unparalleled threat to public health; an incomparable challenge to international development and global security. One hesitates to add another appellation to the list. But the fact remains that in the United States and in many other nations of the world, HIV/AIDS has proven to be an unprecedented catalyst to the development of important scientific, technical, and policy advances.

Certainly, the measure of knowledge and positive experience that has come from this epidemic is small in comparison to the staggering worldwide cost of suffering and death caused by HIV. Nevertheless, what we have learned in over two decades of dealing with this virus is significant—not only because the knowledge is hard won but also because the information we have amassed about HIV/AIDS can be applied for the benefit of future generations in combating this epidemic and other, related challenges to health around the globe.

Among the most obvious advances are those in antiretroviral therapeutics. Although we are still far from a cure, the advent of highly effective, combination antiretroviral therapy has had the phenomenal and well-publicized effect of decreasing AIDS incidence and AIDS deaths in the United States and in several European countries. Equally stunning, although perhaps not as well recognized by the general public, are the myriad accomplishments in a broad range of AIDS-related scientific disciplines, including immunology, virology, and genetics. Research into the natural history and pathogenesis of HIV has increased our understanding of the mechanisms by which viral and cell factors control gene expression. An increased understanding of how cells of the human immune system communicate with one another has profound implications for the large variety of illnesses known as "autoimmune" diseases. From our collective efforts to diagnose and treat HIV infection, inroads have been made into the understanding and treatment of scores of medical conditions in addition to HIV.

Not all of the important advances in HIV/AIDS science have been medical. This disease, known for its cruel ability to rob its victims of vitality and productivity, has done much to energize the field of public health. In response to the epidemic, public health theory and practice have undergone a substantial evolution, which is the subject of this text.

Public health, with its focus on communities and populations, promotes health and protects against disease by assuring conditions in which people can be healthy. This broad mission is accomplished through three "core" functions: assessing the health of communities and populations at risk; formulating sound public policies to address health threats; and assuring that all populations have access to needed health care and prevention services. As this book explains, advances in public health techniques and strategies (e.g., in monitoring health events, developing public policy, setting funding priorities, mobilizing communities, etc.) all owe a substantial debt to those who have adapted, refined, and extended these techniques and strategies in response to HIV/AIDS.

Although the examples provided in this text are specific to the HIV/AIDS experience, their potential application to other public health problems is recognized and discussed. For instance, a community-based, priority-setting process developed to direct public health HIV prevention funds, described in Chapter 3, could be adapted by communities to determine other important health priorities, such as environmental health priorities. And antidiscrimination legislation passed in response to HIV/AIDS provides a useful framework for addressing related issues that are currently arising in the realm of human genetics testing. Advances in surveillance techniques, including the development of surrogate measures of HIV incidence (see "detuned" assay in Chapter 2) can be applied to monitoring other infectious diseases.

This book offers detailed analyses from experts across the various disciplines that constitute public health. The preponderance of examples reflects the U.S. experience, although relevant examples from other countries are cited and an entire chapter is devoted to the evolving impact of HIV/AIDS on global health and development. Students and teachers of public health and preventive medicine will find in this comprehensive volume a singular, albeit practical, encapsulation of each of the key dimensions of current public health science and practice. As such, this volume provides a much-needed context for ongoing discussions of public health infrastructure and public health workforce development. Likewise, HIV prevention researchers and practitioners will find the information contained in this book useful and highly relevant, as it provides an up-to-date summary of advances in HIV/AIDS policy, program, and behavioral research.

Not all of AIDS' lessons have been positive, of course. Nor has triumph been the inevitable outcome of each human–viral interaction. HIV/AIDS is truly a tragedy of global dimensions, and its toll can never be viewed as less than devastating. But sobering though its effects are, we cannot ignore the fact that the many lessons learned through the HIV/AIDS experience have acted as a catalyst to public health in the development of new approaches to assessment, policy development, and assurance. There will be a day in the future when, if not gone, HIV/AIDS will no longer be the global threat that it is at this point in human history. But its important public health legacy will remain with us forever.

Atlanta, Georgia   R.O.V.

Contents

Contributors

RONALD BAYER, Ph.D.
Joseph L. Mailman School of Public Health
Columbia University
New York, New York

JAMES W. BUEHLER, M.D.
Center for Public Health Preparedness
*   and Research*
Rollins School of Public Health
Emory University
Atlanta, Georgia

SCOTT BURRIS, J.D.
James E. Beasley School of Law
Temple University
Philadelphia, Pennsylvania

WILLARD CATES, JR., M.D., M.P.H.
Family Health International
Research Triangle Park, North Carolina

JAMES W. CURRAN, M.D., M.P.H.
Rollins School of Public Health
Emory University
Atlanta, Georgia

LAWRENCE O. GOSTIN, J.D., L.L.D.
Georgetown University/Johns Hopkins
*   University*
Washington, D.C.

MARY E. GUINAN, M.D., Ph.D.
Nevada Public Health Foundation
Carson City, Nevada

DAVID R. HOLTGRAVE, Ph.D.
Emory Center for AIDS Research
Rollins School of Public Health
Emory University
Atlanta, Georgia

PETER LAMPTEY, M.D., Dr.P.H.
Institute for HIV/AIDS
Family Health International
Arlington, Virginia

JEFFREY LEVI, Ph.D.
*George Washington School of Public
    Health and Health Services
Washington, D.C.*

LAURA C. LEVITON, M.A., Ph.D.
*Robert Wood Johnson Foundation
Princeton, New Jersey*

ROBERT M. MALOW, Ph.D.
*Department of Psychiatry and
    Behavioral Sciences
University of Miami School of Medicine
Miami, Florida*

ANN O'LEARY, Ph.D.
*Division of HIV/AIDS Prevention:
    Intervention Research and Support
National Center for HIV, STD,
    and TB Prevention
Centers for Disease Control and Prevention
Atlanta, Georgia*

KRISTEN RUCKSTUHL, M.A.
*Family Health International
Arlington, Virginia*

RONALD O. VALDISERRI, M.D., M.P.H.
*National Center for HIV, STD,
    and TB Prevention
Centers for Disease Control and
    Prevention
Atlanta, Georgia*

LINDA WRIGHT-DEAGÜERO, Ph.D.,
    M.P.H.
*Division of HIV/AIDS Prevention:
    Intervention Research and Support
National Center for HIV, STD, and
    TB Prevention
Centers for Disease Control and
    Prevention
Atlanta, Georgia*

Dawning Answers

1

HIV/AIDS in Historical Profile

RONALD O. VALDISERRI

That epidemics of infectious disease leave behind their footprints in history is not a novel observation. Some of humanity's most intriguing episodes document the unexpected effects of human–microbial interaction. A significant consequence of the Black Death among European bourgeoisie, it has been argued, was a new conception of time, a pronounced sense of urgency that was manifest in longer working days, night work, and the increasing popularity of clocks and time-keeping bell chimes (1). Cortez's victory over the Aztecs was almost certainly facilitated by smallpox carried to the New World by the conquistadors who, unlike the hapless Aztecs, were largely immune (2). And after an aggressive 1,250 square mile advance, which brought German artillery within striking range of Paris, the offensive was halted in July 1918, when thousands of German soldiers succumbed to influenza, giving Allied forces the opportunity to replenish their troops and lead a counteroffensive that eventually ended the war (3).

McNeill's description of infectious disease as a "fundamental parameter and determinant of human history" (4) certainly applies to AIDS, the acquired immunodeficiency syndrome. Human immunodeficiency virus (HIV), the cause of AIDS, has a common heritage with past infectious disease epidemics in its ability to influence the way that we live our lives and the questions we ask about our world—even how we craft our laws and invest our public resources.

More specifically, the central premise of this book is that among the many consequences of the HIV/AIDS epidemic have been substantial and ongoing changes in public health theory and practice—both domestically and internationally. Clearly, societal responses to HIV/AIDS have not always been constructive, nor are all of the lessons learned necessarily positive. These limitations notwithstanding, the global epidemic of HIV/AIDS is undeniably a significant public health event that will leave its mark on approaches and responses to other public health challenges well into the next century.

Our nation's history provides examples of how infectious disease epidemics of the past have influenced public health—in terms of both their effect on the development of scientific knowledge and in their ability to shape public opinions, values, and actions. In response to the 1866–1867 cholera epidemic, a number of American cities, including Chicago, St. Louis, and Cincinnati, established standing, independent health boards. Before that time, health matters "were usually handled through city councils and police departments or through volunteer health officials without tangible authority" (5). The spread of yellow fever from New Orleans upward into the Mississippi Valley in 1878 "mobilized widespread support for a national quarantine system" (6). More recently, the increasing incidence of polio in the 1950s galvanized public support for a large, multistate study of the effectiveness of gamma globulin as a polio preventive (7). Although that particular study failed to demonstrate efficacy, continued public concern about epidemic polio helped to fuel the eventual development of an effective vaccine (7).

Admittedly, as we enter a new century, humanity has not concluded its dealings with HIV/AIDS. While effective HIV treatment and prevention strategies exist, at the time of this writing, there is neither a cure nor an effective vaccine for HIV infection. And the epidemic continues to spread. At the end of 2000 it was estimated that over 36 million persons, globally, were living with HIV/AIDS, more than 5 million having become newly infected in 2000 alone (8). In the same time period in the United States, an estimated 800,000 to 900,000 persons were living with HIV/AIDS, with approximately 40,000 additional Americans becoming newly infected each year (9). No one disputes that the history of HIV/AIDS is still unfolding.

To what end, then, is a historical profile? As Berridge explains in the introduction to her volume on AIDS and contemporary history, there are three broad functions of historical policy writing: historical analysis to inform current policy development or to forecast the future; analysis of past events using particular theoretical models, "without specific current policy intent"; and re-creating the past for its own sake—what she describes as "academic 'voyeurism'" (10). It is the first of these functions that will predominate throughout this book—namely: to describe and place in context a variety of changes in public health theory and practice that are related, either wholly or in large part, to the unfolding HIV/AIDS epidemic and to exemplify and extrapolate their application to other important public health problems. In our discussion, we will adopt the Institute of Medicine's definition of public health's mission as "fulfilling society's interest in assuring conditions in which people can be healthy" (11). To prepare for this discussion, we provide a general historical review of the HIV/AIDS epidemic and highlight major milestones.

An Epidemic Comes to Light

Based on molecular epidemiologic studies, scientists now believe that HIV was originally a simian virus that was somehow transmitted to human hosts—a zoonotic infection (12). Strains of immunodeficiency virus that were transmitted from chimpanzees to humans have come to be known as HIV-1 and those that were transmitted to humans from sooty mangabeys are known as HIV-2 (12,13). Precisely how this happened will remain conjecture, but a plausible scenario can be constructed around exposure to infected simian blood during the process of butchering and preparing "bush meat" for consumption—a not uncommon practice in sub-Saharan Africa (14,15). Next, a variety of demographic, social, and situational circumstances turned what was likely sporadic episodes of "dead-end" human to human viral transmission into rapid and widespread infection (14). In the Western world, the global epidemic of HIV came to light in early June 1981 (16).

On June 5, 1981, the Centers for Disease Control and Prevention (CDC) reported on five previously healthy, homosexual men who had been treated for biopsy-proven *Pneumocystis carinii* pneumonia (PCP) (16). The cluster of cases was noteworthy because the five men had no clinically apparent underlying immunodeficiency and, as the report stated, PCP in the United States "is almost exclusively limited to severely immunosuppressed patients" (16) . The next month CDC reported that twenty-six homosexual men from New York City and California had been diagnosed with Kaposi's sarcoma (KS), a rare, vascular malignancy typically seen in elderly men (17). By the end of August 1981, some 108 Americans had been reported with either PCP or KS, or both; all but one were men, nearly three-quarters were white, and nearly 90 percent of the men were homosexual or bisexual (18).

Due to its initial appearance in gay men, the mysterious condition was unofficially called "GRID," or gay-related immune deficiency. However, it soon became apparent that this condition was not limited to gay men. Following the first case reports, unexplained cellular immunodeficiency and accompanying opportunistic infections were reported among heterosexual men and women (19), injecting drug users (19), Haitian men and women residing in the United States (20), persons with hemophilia A (21), a 20-month-old infant who had been multiply transfused following birth (22), and four infants born to mothers who themselves had the condition or were at increased risk for it (23). With mounting evidence that some heretofore undescribed agent was being transmitted sexually and through exposure to blood, that it was causing previously healthy persons to develop diseases typically associated with profound immunodeficiency, the new condition was named the acquired immune deficiency syndrome (24).

Following the U.S. reports, published accounts of AIDS-like illnesses occurring among African patients hospitalized in Europe (25,26,27), as well as among African nationals (28), began to appear. Africans with AIDS had the same immunologic abnormalities observed in Americans and Europeans with the disease (28). Unlike their counterparts from the industrialized world, however, where persons with AIDS were predominantly male, African AIDS cases were equally distributed among men and women. And there was no evidence of homosexuality or injecting drug use among Africans with the condition (29).

In March 1983, the U.S. Public Health Service issued recommendations for the prevention of AIDS (30); earlier published "precautions" had been limited to hospital and laboratory workers (31). The 1983 recommendations stated that, while the cause of AIDS was unknown, sexual contact with persons known or suspected to have AIDS should be avoided (30). Also, members of groups at increased risk for AIDS were urged to refrain from donating plasma or blood (30). Two months later, in May 1983, researchers from the Institute Pasteur in Paris reported the isolation of a T-lymphotropic retrovirus, named lymphadenopathy-associated virus (LAV), from a gay man with diffuse, generalized lymphadenopathy—a clinically recognized precursor of AIDS (32). One year later, researchers from the U.S. National Cancer Institute reported the isolation of a morphologically similar T-lymphotropic virus (HTLV-III) from the lymphocytes of twenty-six of seventy-two patients with AIDS and from eighteen of twenty-one patients with conditions that were considered to be clinical precursors of AIDS (33). The high prevalence of circulating antibodies to HTLV-III/LAV (as the virus was then called) among homosexual men with lymphadenopathy, injecting drug users, and persons with hemophilia A added substantially to the supposition that HTLV-III/LAV was the cause of AIDS (34). However, at the time, the prognostic implications of a positive HTLV-III/LAV test were unknown; it was unclear whether a positive test represented current infection or immunity (34).

Early Public Indifference

Several analyses posit that the initial occurrence of this dread new disease among socially stigmatized groups—homosexuals and injecting drug users—was largely responsible for an inadequate response to the burgeoning epidemic in both the public and private sectors (35,36,37,38). Media analysts have juxtaposed the extensive media coverage garnered by the 1976 Legionnaires' disease outbreak in Philadelphia to the limited national coverage received by AIDS in its early years.

This, despite the fact that AIDS affected more people and had a substantially higher mortality rate than Legionnaire's disease (35,36). Much is also made of the fact that the *New York Times*, the nation's newspaper of record, did not publish a front-page story on AIDS until May 25, 1983—nearly two years after the epidemic was first recognized (35).

Approximately a year after the initial cases of AIDS had been reported, the first "mainstream" magazine in America ran an article about AIDS, on May 31, 1982 (39). That the article was entitled "The Gay Plague" was telling, for it underscored the lens through which most Americans viewed the epidemic—if they were cognizant of it at all. Although AIDS among heterosexuals had been described early on in the United States (19), and the AIDS epidemic in Africa was almost exclusively heterosexual, the preponderance of homosexual men comprising the U.S. epidemic left those citizens who were aware of AIDS feeling far removed from its threat for much of the first decade of the epidemic.

Inadequate Response

Mainstream America's lack of familiarity with two largely hidden subcultures (i.e., gay men and injecting drug users) contributed to the public's subsequent lack of identification with the risks of AIDS. But unawareness, by itself, doesn't fully explain society's early response to the epidemic. Other factors were at play. Because homosexuality and injecting drug use are both highly stigmatized behaviors, many officials and policy-makers were uncomfortable confronting these subjects in an open manner. Some even viewed the syndrome along moralistic lines, blaming the persons who became infected through sex and drug use, while sympathizing with those infected in utero or through exposure to contaminated blood transfusions. In this regard, reactions to AIDS were reminiscent of our nation's historical response to another sexually transmitted disease, syphilis. In the early twentieth century, physicians referred to the wives and children of infected men as the "innocent victims" of syphilis (40); a similar judgmental distinction would be applied some eighty years later in regard to AIDS (41).

Epidemiologic circumstances may also have helped minimize the perceived threat of AIDS, thus contributing to its initial, tepid public response. During its early years in the United States, AIDS was highly concentrated in the coastal urban areas (42); other parts of the nation, especially interior states and rural areas, may have underestimated the potential impact of AIDS on their own jurisdictions. Even within the same geographic area, AIDS risk could vary substantially. In the first decade of the epidemic, researchers estimating the risk of heterosexual transmission hypothesized tremendous variations in risk per act of intercourse, ranging from 1 in 500 to 1 in 5 million, depending on partner status (43). Given the difficulties that most people have thinking in terms of probabilities (44), disparate estimates such as these may have served to confuse the public, further diminishing perceptions of risk, especially among heterosexuals.

Perhaps the greatest epidemiological impediment to an early, aggressive response to AIDS was an underestimation of the magnitude of the epidemic (45). To identify new cases and determine the extent of the epidemic, the first AIDS case definition was published in September 1982 (24); periodic revisions to the surveillance case definition would be made over time, reflecting advances in clinical and laboratory science and progress in understanding the natural history and pathogenesis of the disease (46). However, it wasn't until April 1984 that a longitudinal natural history study of AIDS was funded in the United States (47), and some three years following before the study began to yield results (48). Further, tests to detect circulating antibodies to HTLV-III/LAV were not available until March 1985 (49). Therefore, several years passed between the first observation of the AIDS epidemic and an informed estimate of its potential magnitude.

In June 1986, the U.S. Public Health Service estimated that between 1 and 1.5 million Americans were infected with HTLV-III/LAV and that 20 to 30 percent of those persons would eventually go on to develop AIDS (50). Although estimates of infected Americans made at the end of the century would be somewhat smaller, in the range of 800,000 to 900,000 (9), we now know that nearly all persons infected with HIV will go on to experience a reduction in CD4+ cells, eventually followed by symptomatic disease (51).

A detailed policy analysis of the first five years of the AIDS epidemic, published in the late 1980s, added organizational structures and processes to the list of variables responsible for "problems in responding to the AIDS emergency" (52). Panem observed that the "start of the epidemic coincided with a time when the overriding federal budgetary concern was a reduction of the federal deficit, to be achieved by reducing spending for domestic programs" (53). Along with a "lack of available financial resources and flexible budget authority" at the federal level, she cited the absence of a formal "mechanism to coordinate diverse health activities during an emergency" and "neglect of strategic planning" in response to the novel challenges posed by the AIDS epidemic (52).

Five years into the epidemic, when the National Academy of Sciences (NAS) and the Institute of Medicine (IOM) published a report reviewing the public- and private-sector response to AIDS, they concluded that expenditures for education and other public health measures were "inadequate" (45). The committee recommended expanding existing prevention efforts, improving the provision and financing of medical care for persons with AIDS, increasing biomedical and behavioral research efforts, and affirming a national commitment to the control of AIDS. At the time, the IOM committee recommended that the federal government invest $1 billion annually into AIDS-related research and that there be "a significant federal contribution toward the $1 billion annually required for the total costs of education and public health measures" (45). Actual Public Health Service funding for AIDS in 1985 was approximately $118 million dollars, with about 28 percent of the funds targeted toward prevention activities and 54 percent supporting research (53).

Affected Communities' Reaction

One of the earliest, and most enduring, hallmarks of the AIDS epidemic has been the response of affected communities. In the early 1980s, the first AIDS community-based organizations (CBOs) were founded in the United States; pre-eminent examples include the Gay Men's Health Crisis in New York City, the AIDS Project Los Angeles, and the San Francisco AIDS Foundation (54,55). Many of the earliest AIDS CBOs were founded by members of the gay community. Horrified by the mounting death toll and angry about public indifference, gay community activists took steps to organize services for those with AIDS, deliver prevention education, challenge discrimination against people with AIDS, and mobilize broader support to address the epidemic (38).

A "strong group identity" (54) and a high level of organization within many communities of gay men helped to facilitate a rapid response to the emerging epidemic. Other affected populations, including injection drug users (IDUs) and racial and ethnic minorities, also responded to the threat of AIDS by developing or strengthening community-based efforts to provide prevention and care services (56). Yet, even before the onset of AIDS, economically disadvantaged racial and ethnic minority communities faced a multiplicity of other "survival" issues (57), including substandard housing and inadequate municipal services (58), which impeded their ability to mount a rapid and comprehensive community response during the early years of the AIDS epidemic.

Expanded Community Role

As pointed out by Freudenberg and Zimmerman, "community mobilization against threats to health did not . . . begin with AIDS"; historically, community organizations have played "an active role in combating tuberculosis, infant mortality, and sexually transmitted diseases," among others (59). Furthermore, the involvement of non-governmental organizations (NGOs) in public health matters (60) is entirely consistent with the definition that public health is what "we, as a society, do collectively to assure the conditions in which people can be healthy" (11). However, this analyst concurs with Freudenberg and Zimmerman's observation that "the community response to AIDS prevention and services represented a qualitatively different level of involvement than previous reactions to other health conditions" (59). Specifically, not only were AIDS CBOs committed to the delivery of needed prevention and care services, but also the epidemic saw them becoming frequently and prominently involved in the three core public health functions of assessment, assurance, and policy development—activities that typically fall within the purview of government organizations (11).

For example, to better assess the prevention needs of gay men, in 1984 the San Francisco AIDS Foundation commissioned a random, probability-based survey of 500 self-identified gay and bisexual men from the city and county of San Francisco (61). The survey collected detailed information on sexual practices, perceived risk of AIDS, community norms related to sexual risk, and credible sources of AIDS information. Results of this assessment were used to develop an AIDS prevention campaign that stressed the social acceptability of safe sex rather than only the risks of unsafe practices (62).

An excellent example of guaranteeing necessary health services—the assurance function—is provided by the Health Crisis Network from Miami Florida. This CBO developed a "transportable" training package, including videotaped vignettes, as a means of ensuring the high quality of counseling provided by nonprofessional volunteers who facilitated risk-reduction discussions among groups of gay men (63). The Gay Men's Health Crisis (GMHC) in New York City provides another example of the assurance function. GMHC teamed up with the New York City Department of Mental Health and an academic medical center to form a training and service network to ensure that New York's community of mental health providers had the skills required to care for persons with AIDS (PWAs), those at risk for the disease, loved ones of PWAs, and other caregivers (64).

Sound public health policy development calls for the use of scientific knowledge in decision making, as well as decisive, strategic leadership—often in the face of strong opposing views. Of the various examples of non-governmental organizations embracing the traditional government role of public health policy development in response to the AIDS epidemic, none is more compelling than the issue of providing access to sterile injection equipment for active injection drug users as a strategy to reduce viral transmission.

The first organized needle exchange project was started in 1984, in Amsterdam, by an association of drug users (the Junkies' Union); they sought to reduce the spread of hepatitis B virus and prevent AIDS among IDUs (65). Although pragmatic U.S. public health leaders had proposed the distribution of clean needles to IDUs as an anti-AIDS measure as early as 1985 (66), the issue of access to sterile injection equipment was, and remains, highly controversial. Opposition often centers on fears that needle exchange programs (NEPs) will encourage drug use (67). Many community leaders, especially from racial and ethnic minority communities, are opposed to NEPs because they consider them to be an inadequate (and potentially lethal) alternative to providing sufficient substance abuse prevention and treatment services to communities in need (67). Several NEPs that had been "strongly supported by city public health departments" were successfully blocked because of strong community opposition (68).

In New York, on August 11, 1988, the state granted a waiver, under its needle prescription statute, to the New York City Health Department to conduct a pilot NEP (68), slated to provide a proposed 6,000 injectors with up to five sterile syringes per visit to any of four community-based health centers in the New York City area (69). The New York NEP was the "first government approved, sponsored, and funded needle exchange" in the United States (69). However, several months would pass before a "scaled-down" version of the original proposal was actually implemented, involving only 200 injectors who could receive a single clean syringe by visiting "an old x-ray room at the central offices of the New York City Department of Health" (69). Some fourteen months later, in January 1990, the pilot program was terminated when a new mayor took office (69).

Before the waiver was approved, a Brooklyn-based CBO, the Association for Drug Abuse Prevention and Treatment (ADAPT) (56), defied state law and began distributing sterile needles and syringes in January 1988 (66). Frustrated by mounting AIDS cases among injecting drug users and recognizing that many IDUs were unwilling or unable to stop their drug use, ADAPT took this bold step "to challenge the state in the name of public health" (70). According to Anderson's analysis of New York's needle exchange pilot, this action by ADAPT "forced the issue" and helped to move forward state administrative approval of a clinical trial of needle and syringe distribution (71).

The American Foundation for AIDS Research (AmFAR), a nonprofit organization devoted to AIDS research, prevention, treatment education, and the advocacy of sound AIDS-related public policy, has been extremely active in policy development on the subject of access to sterile injection equipment for IDUs. Since 1988, AmFAR has invested nearly $4 million to support the scientific evaluation of needle exchange programs (72). Academic researchers receiving AmFAR funding conducted an analysis of IDUs participating in syringe exchange programs versus nonparticipants and found an "individual level protective effect against HIV infection associated with participation in a syringe exchange programme" (73). Using federal funds to support needle exchange programs has been banned by U.S. law since 1988 (74), and the ban remains in place at the time of this writing. But, there is no doubt that non-governmental organizations, through their expanded role in policy development (75), will continue to vivify the public dialogue on this important and controversial prevention topic.

Increasing AIDS Awareness

In July 1985, the famous American film star Rock Hudson announced that he had AIDS (37). Mr. Hudson's disclosure and subsequent death on October 2, 1985, substantially heightened "mainstream" public awareness of the burgeoning epidemic (37). In the interval between Hudson's disclosure and the end of

1985, print media coverage of AIDS increased 270 percent; substantial increases in broadcast coverage were also observed (76).

Although increased AIDS awareness ultimately helped to encourage public funding for the new disease, it also triggered anxiety about the risk of acquiring the virus, "verging on hysteria in some parts of the country" (77). Unfounded fears of casual transmission were evident in a poll taken in the mid-1980s: 47 percent of American adults thought that AIDS could be contracted by sharing a drinking glass, and 28 percent believed the disease could be "picked up from a toilet seat" (77). In 1985, at an elementary school in Queens, New York, 944 of 1,100 students failed to show up for the beginning of the fall term when it was learned that an unidentified second-grader with AIDS was to be enrolled in one of the city's 622 elementary schools (77). Unrealistic fears of transmission via casual contact served to further increase the stigma already associated with AIDS as a result of its connection to the socially disapproved behaviors of homosexuality and drug use (78).

Less touted by the popular media, another significant milestone in the AIDS epidemic occurred the same year as Mr. Hudson's revelation. On March 2, 1985, the Food and Drug Administration (FDA) licensed an enzyme-linked immunosorbent assay (ELISA) test to detect antibodies to HTLV-III/LAV (49). The U.S. Public Health Service issued provisional recommendations on how the new test should be used to screen blood and plasma collected for the purpose of transfusion, strongly emphasizing the importance of confidentiality and recognizing that "disclosure of information for purposes other than medical or public health could lead to serious consequences for the individual" (79).

Testing for Viral Antibodies

Serologic testing for HTLV-III/LAV antibodies eventually negated the risk of acquiring AIDS as a result of blood transfusion—at least in those countries whose health-care systems had resource enough to conduct routine screening of donor units. Less than five months after the test was introduced, it was estimated that as many as 1,000 potentially infectious units of blood had been removed from the U.S. blood supply (80). The new test for HTLV-III/LAV also improved the specificity of the case definition used for national AIDS reporting (81), thus enhancing public health's ability to monitor the epidemic. Another potential benefit was the test's ability to reveal to at-risk persons whether they had actually been infected with the virus—information that could help inform both prevention and medical decision making. For example, the test made it possible for women of reproductive age who were at behavioral risk for AIDS (e.g., partners of IDUs) to learn whether they had been infected with HTLV-III/LAV, thereby providing specific information for their reproductive decision making (82). From a research perspective, the test enabled the study of disease progression among persons who were found to be infected but had not yet manifested any signs or symptoms of AIDS.

Not all of the outcomes of this technological advance were positive. At an individual level, uncertainty about the prognostic value of a positive test result was a disincentive to seeking the test for many "high-risk" persons who suspected they had been exposed to the virus. When a group of scientific experts met in July 1986 to consider, among other things, "How should a positive HIV antibody test be interpreted?", they concluded "we cannot precisely predict who among persons with antibody positivity will be ill or fatally ill in the future and it is not possible at present to prevent such outcomes" (83). Two years would intervene between the licensure of the HTLV-III/LAV test and the FDA's approval of the first antiretroviral treatment shown to prolong survival in persons with AIDS (84). A client-level brochure produced in 1986 by the National Gay Rights Advocates organization reflected a similar sentiment: "The HTLV-III antibody test doesn't tell if you have or will develop AIDS" (85). And when 9 percent of a cohort of gay and bisexual men enrolled in a federally funded natural history study of AIDS declined to learn their antibody status, the most frequently cited reason the men gave for not wanting to learn test results was "because the test is not predictive of AIDS" (86).

Over time, as the natural history of AIDS came to light, uncertainty about the prognostic implications of a positive test would be resolved, and treatment advances would increase the medical benefits of early diagnosis. Slower to dissipate was the firmly held conviction of those who saw widespread screening, including mandatory testing of high-risk groups, as a public health panacea for containing the spread of this dread virus. The belief that large-scale testing would stop the spread of AIDS had its roots in the nation's experience with another major sexually transmitted disease epidemic—syphilis. In 1937, Surgeon General Thomas Parran advocated that syphilis could be "conquered" in the United States by aggressive case finding, prompt treatment, identification and treatment of the patient's sexual partners, public education, and mandatory premarital and prenatal blood testing (87). But unlike the situation with AIDS in the late 1980s, individuals found to be infected with syphilis in the 1930s could be treated and rendered noninfectious (88). Yet, even at the time of Parran's campaign, "mandatory premarital serologies never proved to be a particularly effective mechanism for finding new cases of syphilis" (89).

After the U.S. Department of Defense began screening all military applicants for antibodies to HTLV-III/LAV in late 1985, other proposals surfaced for mandatory testing programs (88). For the most part, the public health community agreed that there was little public health benefit to be obtained from mandatory screening, whether for the general population or for high-risk population subgroups (90,91). Commonly cited by public health experts was the concern that mandatory testing might drive high-risk people away from the very public health system that was attempting to reach them and their partners with accurate AIDS information (91,92). With the notable exception of recommending that all organ, tissue, and semen donors be tested for antibodies to HTLV-III/LAV (93) and that all donated blood and plasma be screened for HTLV-III/LAV antibodies (79), the U.S. Public Health Service did not recommend mandatory testing. Instead, recommendations to reduce sexual, parenteral, and perinatal transmission of the virus all stressed the importance of voluntary, confidential testing (82,94).

Undesirable Social Responses

By the time the HTLV-III/LAV antibody test began to move into clinical and public health practice, a variety of scientific evaluations had clearly confirmed that HTLV-III/LAV could be transmitted sexually, parenterally (i.e., through exposure to infected blood), and perinatally (95)—that is, it was not a virus transmitted through casual exposures or normal day-to-day interactions (96,97). As such, official U.S. Public Health Service recommendations concerning the potential transmission of the virus in health-care and school settings indicated that routine serologic testing of patients (98) and mandatory testing of schoolchildren (99) were not recommended as prevention strategies. Nevertheless, mounting alarm over this incurable disease continued to fuel exaggerated fears of transmission—another similarity between the social response to AIDS and the reaction to syphilis in the early twentieth century (87).

Sadly, instances of discrimination in employment, housing, medical care, public accommodations, and education against persons with AIDS began to occur very early in the epidemic (100,101)—well before the licensure of a test for HTLV-III/LAV antibodies. However, with the development of a test capable of identifying persons who had been infected, before they manifested signs or symptoms of AIDS, concerns about potential discrimination broadened.

The first Presidential Commission on Human Immunodeficiency Virus (as the virus had, by then, come to be known) issued its report to President Ronald Reagan in June 1988; they observed that "HIV-related discrimination is impairing this nation's ability to limit the spread of the epidemic" and called on the president to "issue an executive order banning discrimination on the basis of handicap with HIV infection included as a handicapping condition" (102). The World Health Organization took a similar position, calling on all member states "to protect the human rights and dignity of HIV-infected people and people with AIDS . . . and to avoid discriminatory action against and stigmatization of them in the provision of services, employment, and travel" (103).

According to Gostin, antidiscrimination legislation protecting persons with communicable diseases did not emerge until "remarkably recently" in U.S. legislative history (100). Indubitably, the AIDS epidemic played a major role in sensitizing policy-makers to issues of stigma and discrimination related to infectious diseases (41). In 1990, when the Americans with Disabilities Act (ADA) was signed into law, making discrimination on the basis of disability unlawful, it included AIDS as a disability (104). The ADA has been hailed as a "historic civil-rights law" protecting disabled Americans from discrimination that results from "fear and prejudice" (104). Supplementing the protection provided by the ADA, "state laws frequently prohibit disability discrimination and apply to some employers and others not regulated by federal law" (105).

The HIV/AIDS epidemic has advanced our concepts of "discrimination" and "disability" to include infectious diseases. More broadly, the epidemic has pointed out the integral relationship between public health goals and human rights, advancing the concept that "when human rights are protected, fewer people become infected and those living with HIV/AIDS and their families can better cope with HIV/AIDS" (106).

Caring for the Sick

The impact of AIDS on the planning, delivery, and financing of health-care services is an area deserving of special attention and will be addressed in subsequent chapters of this book. In the United States, scarcely a dimension of health-care—from the design and development of clinical trials, to health-care worker recruitment and training—has remained untouched by the epidemic. Early analyses of AIDS health policy identified resource constraints as significant barriers to the development of comprehensive care services—especially in a health-care environment of pervasive "cost-containment" (107). In the late 1980s, one commentator observed that the United States was particularly ill-equipped to deal with the burgeoning medical needs of persons with AIDS because of its "dependency on tertiary care hospitals, ultraspecialization, and the fragility of health-care financing mechanisms" (108).

As with many dimensions of the epidemic, however, challenge spurred innovation. Ambulatory and in-patient services created for AIDS patients in San Francisco, which stressed multidisciplinary integration and close coordination with community providers, were considered models of excellence and were emulated elsewhere in the United States (109). Community-based organizations played a vital role in delivering health-care to persons with AIDS and symptomatic HIV disease, and they continue to do so. A 1989 case study of Los Angeles, Miami, New York, and San Francisco demonstrated that large CBOs in these four communities were providing many needed out-of-hospital services to persons with AIDS, including home care (110).

Innovations notwithstanding, resources remained a significant barrier to caring for those with HIV disease, especially in low-income communities. Even in communities with large, well-managed CBOs, concerns were raised about the long-term viability of supporting vital client services through volunteer labor and private charity (55). And as the epidemic advanced, the public health-care sector began to show signs of strain. Between 1983 and 1988, hospitalizations of patients with a diagnosis of HIV increased twenty-six-fold in the United States (111), and a 1987 U.S. hospital survey suggested that hospitals serving large numbers of low-income AIDS patients were "encountering moderate to severe financial shortfalls" (112).

In the developing world, the impact of HIV/AIDS on the health-care sector has been even more pronounced. In 1995, the World Bank estimated that the percentage of hospital beds occupied by HIV-positive patients was 50 percent or more in Chiang Mai, Thailand; Kinshasa, Congo DR; Kigali, Rwanda; Kampala, Uganda; and Bujumbura, Burundi (113). AIDS increased demand for health-care, especially among "prime age adults" (i.e., 15 to 50 years old), while at the same time reducing the supply of available health-care; HIV-negative persons were being "crowded-out" of the health-care sector by the increasing demands of HIV/AIDS (113). As a result of AIDS, health-care in developing nations has become more scarce and more expensive and national health-care expenditures rose—especially in the poorest countries with the largest epidemics (113).

After several years of experience dealing with persons with symptomatic HIV disease, a consensus began to develop among providers in the United States, embracing the need for "a comprehensive, coordinated continuum of hospital and community-based services" in caring for persons with HIV/AIDS (114). This consensus, coupled with strong, ongoing advocacy from AIDS service organizations and the gay community, resulted in the passage of the Ryan White Comprehensive AIDS Resources Emergency (CARE) Act of 1990 (115). Signed into law by President George H.W. Bush on August 18, 1990, this law authorized funding for emergency assistance to metropolitan areas that were hit hardest by the epidemic and grant programs to states for the provision of community-based HIV-related care and services (116).

The CARE act serves an important "safety net" function by providing a broad range of services to HIV-infected persons who are poor and underinsured (117). However, as discussed in Chapter 6, the implementation of CARE has done much to highlight problems in the U.S. health-care system—especially weaknesses related to access, financing, and administrative inefficiencies, including multiple, complex funding streams (118). As a result of the AIDS epidemic, U.S. policy-makers have been forced to confront cross-cutting health-care delivery issues such as financing prevention services, reducing variation in health-care eligibility and benefits across states, enhancing coordination of discrete funding streams and categorical services, and addressing the cost of prescription drugs (119). And, while far from resolution, continued innovations in the delivery of care to people with HIV may result in improvements in access for others who are "dependent upon the publicly financed safety net for their health-care" (118).

Internationally, many of the countries where HIV/AIDS is most severe can ill afford to provide adequate therapies for their citizens. In sub-Saharan Africa, where 70 percent of the world's HIV infected persons live (8), average per capita health expenditures range from $10 to $200, far below the cost of antiretroviral therapy and treatments for several of the more common opportunistic infections (120). But here, too, the epidemic has generated nontraditional responses. The United Nations is assisting third-world governments in negotiating with pharmaceutical companies for reduced drug pricing to improve access to treatment (121). Brazil has taken the bold step of providing free, state-of-the-art antiretroviral therapy to all persons infected with HIV; many of the drugs used in the Brazilian program are produced as generic formulations in state-run factories (122). And following the 2000 G8 Summit in Okinawa, leaders of the world's richest countries announced their intention to develop a Global Health Fund to mobilize, manage, and disburse hundreds of millions of dollars to bridge funding gaps in HIV/AIDS, tuberculosis, and malaria control (123). Global leaders and international organizations will continue to grapple with the myriad challenges inherent in providing high-quality HIV treatment and care to infected persons throughout the world. Their successes, as well as their failures, will expand and sharpen our shared understanding of the economic, logistical, and ethical dimensions of international health.

Taming the Virus

AIDS has been credited with producing a heightened sensitivity to "emerging" infectious diseases, which is reflected in both our popular and our scientific cultures (124). Humanity's growing awareness of the global effects of emerging infections is due, in part, to the difficulties we've faced in our collective efforts to quash HIV. The virus has not been an easy adversary. After the first U.S. reports of AIDS in 1981, some six years passed before the Food and Drug Administration (FDA) licensed zidovudine (AZT), the first specific treatment proven to be effective against HIV (84).

Clinical trials demonstrated that zidovudine could prolong survival in persons with AIDS (125) and decrease the progression to AIDS among persons with CD4+ lymphocyte counts below 500 cubic millimeters (126,127). Another, extremely important, application of zidovudine was identified in 1994 when a clinical trial demonstrated that the drug could reduce, by nearly two-thirds, the maternal-to-infant transmission of HIV (128,129).

Unfortunately, cumulative clinical experience with zidovudine revealed that its therapeutic effects lessened over time and no demonstrable survival benefit resulted from prolonged therapy in asymptomatic infected persons (130). In response to the limitations of zidovudine monotherapy, researchers began testing combinations of antiretroviral agents, which proved to be superior in terms of immunologic improvement and reductions in viral load (e.g., 131,132,133).

Treatment for HIV disease took a tremendous leap forward in December 1995, when a new class of antiretroviral agents, the protease inhibitors, were introduced into clinical use (134,135). The combination of protease inhibitors with other antiretroviral medications resulted in marked declines in AIDS deaths in those industrialized nations of the world with enough resources to provide these expensive treatments (136,137,138). So impressive were the benefits of the improved therapy that it was dubbed HAART, "highly active antiretroviral therapy," and some commentators prematurely proclaimed the end of the AIDS epidemic (139).

But HAART, too, has come to show its limitations. In addition to its tremendous expense, which puts HAART out of reach of a majority of the world's infected population, the treatment regimen is complex, prone to adherence difficulties, and associated with multiple toxicities (140). Further, the treatment doesn't eradicate HIV; infected cells persist even among HAART-treated persons who have repeatedly undetectable HIV plasma levels (141). And trend data from the late 1990s showing stabilization of declining AIDS deaths in the United States (142) suggest that we may be reaching the limits of extending survival with current therapeutic approaches.

Current limitations notwithstanding, there have been substantial advances in the treatment of HIV infection over the past two decades. And many of the scientific advances in HIV/AIDS therapy will benefit related areas of medicine and public health (143,144). But this is not the only innovation associated with HIV therapeutics. There is another important legacy—namely, the substantive involvement of advocates from affected communities in the development of policies related to HIV drug testing, approval, and pricing has, and will continue to, influence health activism in many other domains (145).

As discussed in Chapter 3, patient advocacy did not begin with AIDS, but it has expanded into new directions as a result of the epidemic. Input from consumers (i.e., persons living with HIV or AIDS and those at high risk for infection) into the design and implementation of clinical research trials (146) has been found to be so helpful that, since 1990, it has become a required component of all federally funded AIDS clinical trials (147). AIDS advocacy groups are also responsible for a more consumer-oriented approach to experimental therapies, including a "faster evaluation of products directed to life-threatening and severely debilitating diseases" (148). And federal funding for HIV prevention (149), care (150), and research activities (151) require that affected communities be involved in the prioritization and allocation of resources. Plainly, HIV/AIDS has had a substantial effect on the role of consumers in health-care policy development.

The World Spins Forward

In his 1993 Pulitzer Prize–winning drama about AIDS, "Angels in America," the playwright Tony Kushner wrote, "This disease will be the death of many of us, but not nearly all. . . . The world only spins forward" (152). Kushner's dialogue is a reminder that some future generation, "happy posterity" in the words of Petrarch, describing a world free of the Black Death (153), will be rid of HIV/AIDS.

Although it is beyond the scope of this chapter to review the accumulated findings from the numerous past and ongoing vaccine trials conducted worldwide, suffice it to say that multiple lines of evidence support the feasibility of eventually developing a safe and effective vaccine against HIV (154). Advances in prevention science have demonstrated that behaviorally based interventions, when appropriately delivered, can result in the reduction or negation of behaviors that lead to HIV transmission (155,156). And there is no reason to doubt the progressive improvement of therapies to treat HIV infection and AIDS. But for the present, no nation on earth has concluded its dealings with this virus. Consequently, the current historical recounting is admittedly a work in progress.

While the definitive chapter on the complete history of HIV/AIDS is yet to be written, our collective experience with this global pandemic has resulted in a wealth of information about its impact on public health theory and practice in a variety of settings and contexts. Given the scope (over two decades and nearly 22 million deaths globally), scale (an estimated 36 million people were living with HIV/AIDS worldwide at the turn of the century), and reach (the effect of HIV/AIDS has been felt socially, scientifically, economically, organizationally, and politically in the United States and throughout the world) of the HIV/AIDS epidemic, it is evident why it has left no dimension of public health untouched. Subsequent chapters will present detailed discussions of HIV/AIDS' influence on essential public health functions, describing how our experiences with this epidemic have and will continue to influence our approaches to other important public health challenges in the United States and elsewhere around the world.

References

1. Gottfried RS: The immediate consequences. In Gottfried RS: *The Black Death: Natural and Human Disaster in Medieval Europe.* Free Press, New York, 1983, pp. 77–103.
2. McNeill WH: Transoceanic exchanges, 1500–1700. In McNeill WH: *Plagues and Peoples.* Doubleday, New York, 1977, pp. 208–241.
3. Oldstone MB: Influenza virus, the plague that may return. In Oldstone MB: *Viruses, Plagues,* and *History.* Oxford University Press, New York, 1998, pp. 172–186.
4. McNeill WH: The ecological impact of medical science and organization since 1700. In McNeill WH: *Plagues and Peoples.* Doubleday, New York, 1977, pp. 242–295.

5. Duffy J: Public health and the Civil War. In Duffy J: *The Sanitarians: A History of American Public Health.* University of Illinois Press, Urbana, 1990, pp. 110–125.

6. Duffy J: Hospitals and the federal government's role in public health. In Duffy J: *The Sanitarians: A History of American Public Health.* University of Illinois Press, Urbana, 1990, pp. 157–174.

7. Etheridge EW: Establishing credibility. In Etheridge EW: *Sentinel for Health: A History of the Centers for Disease Control.* University of California Press, Berkeley, 1992, pp. 67–86.

8. Joint United Nations Programme on HIV/AIDS: *AIDS Epidemic Update.* UNAIDS, Geneva, Switzerland, December 2000.

9. Centers for Disease Control and Prevention: Guidelines for national human immunodeficiency virus case surveillance, including monitoring for human immunodeficiency virus infection and acquired immunodeficiency syndrome. *Morb Mortal Wkly Rep* 48(No. RR-13): 1–31, 1999.

10. Berridge V: Introduction: AIDS and contemporary history. In Berridge V and Strong P (eds.): *AIDS and Contemporary History.* Cambridge University Press, Cambridge, England, 1993, pp. 1–14.

11. Institute of Medicine: Summary and recommendations. In Institute of Medicine: *The Future of Public Health.* National Academy Press, Washington, DC, 1988, pp. 1–18.

12. Hillis DM: Origins of HIV. *Science* 288: 1757–1759, 2000.

13. Korber B, Muldoon M, Theiler J, et al.: Timing of the ancestor of the HIV-1 pandemic strains. *Science* 288: 1789–1796, 2000.

14. Fauci AS: The AIDS epidemic: considerations for the 21st century. *N Engl J Med* 341: 1046–1050, 1999.

15. Chitnis A, Rawls D, and Moore J: Origin of HIV type 1 in colonial French equatorial Africa? *AIDS Res Human Retro* 16: 5–8, 2000.

16. Centers for Disease Control and Prevention: *Pneumocystis* pneumonia. *Morb Mortal Wkly Rep* 30: 250–252, 1981.

17. Centers for Disease Control and Prevention: Kaposi's sarcoma and *Pneumocystis* pneumonia among homosexual men—New York City and California. *Morb Mortal Wkly Rep* 30: 305–308, 1981.

18. Centers for Disease Control and Prevention: Follow-up on Kaposi's sarcoma and *Pneumocystis* pneumonia. *Morb Mortal Wkly Rep* 30: 409–410, 1981.

19. Centers for Disease Control and Prevention: Update on Kaposi's sarcoma and opportunistic infections in previously healthy persons—United States. *Morb Mortal Wkly Rep* 31: 294–301, 1982.

20. Centers for Disease Control and Prevention: Opportunistic infections and Kaposi's sarcoma among Haitians in the United States. *Morb Mortal Wkly Rep* 31: 353–361, 1982.

21. Centers for Disease Control and Prevention: *Pneumocystis* carinii pneumonia among persons with hemophilia A. *Morb Mortal Wkly Rep* 31: 365–367, 1982.

22. Centers for Disease Control and Prevention: Possible transfusion-associated acquired immune deficiency syndrome (AIDS)—California. *Morb Mortal Wkly Rep* 31: 652–654, 1982.

23. Centers for Disease Control and Prevention: Unexplained immunodeficiency and opportunistic infections in infants—New York, New Jersey, California. *Morb Mortal Wkly Rep* 31: 665–667, 1982.

24. Centers for Disease Control and Prevention: Update on acquired immune deficiency syndrome (AIDS)—United States. *Morb Mortal Wkly Rep* 31: 507–514, 1982.

25. Clumeck N, Mascart-Lemone F, de Maulbeuge J, Brenez D, and Marcellis L: Acquired immune deficiency syndrome in black Africans. *Lancet* i: 642, 1983.
26. Brunet JB, Bouvet E, Chaperon J, et al.: Acquired immunodeficiency syndrome in France. *Lancet* i: 700–701, 1983.
27. Clumeck N, Sonnet J, Taelman H, et al.: Acquired immunodeficiency syndrome in African patients. *N Engl J Med* 310: 492–497, 1984.
28. Piot P, Taelman H, Minlangu KB, et al.: Acquired immunodeficiency syndrome in a heterosexual population in Zaire. *Lancet* ii: 65–69, 1984.
29. Quinn TC, Mann JM, Curran JW, and Piot P: AIDS in Africa: an epidemiological paradigm. *Science* 234: 955–963, 1986.
30. Centers for Disease Control and Prevention: Prevention of acquired immune deficiency syndrome (AIDS): report of inter-agency recommendations. *Morb Mortal Wkly Rep* 32: 101–104, 1983.
31. Centers for Disease Control and Prevention: Acquired immune deficiency syndrome (AIDS): precautions for clinical and laboratory staffs. *Morb Mortal Wkly Rep* 31: 577–580, 1982.
32. Barre-Sinoussi F, Chermann JC, Rey F, et al.: Isolation of a T-lymphotropic retrovirus from a patient at risk for acquired immune deficiency syndrome (AIDS). *Science* 220: 868–871, 1983.
33. Gallo RC, Salahuddin SZ, Popovic M, et al.: Frequent detection and isolation of cytopathic retroviruses (HTLV-III) from patients with AIDS and at risk for AIDS. *Science* 224: 500–503, 1984.
34. Centers for Disease Control and Prevention: Antibodies to a retrovirus etiologically associated with acquired immunodeficiency syndrome (AIDS) in populations with increased incidences of the syndrome. *Morb Mortal Wkly Rep* 33: 377–379, 1984.
35. Kinsella J: Sex, death, and good old gray. In Kinsella J: *Covering the Plague: AIDS and the American Media.* Rutgers University Press, New Brunswick, NJ, 1989, pp. 59–86.
36. Public Media Center: *The Impact of Homophobia and Other Social Biases on AIDS.* Public Media Center, San Francisco, 1995.
37. Shilts R: *And the Band Played On: Politics, People, and the AIDS Epidemic.* St. Martin's Press, New York, 1987.
38. Andriote JM: A pox on our house. In Andriote JM: *Victory Deferred: How AIDS Changed Gay Life in America.* University of Chicago Press, Chicago, 1999, pp. 47–82.
39. Ver Meulen M: The gay plague. *New York* 31 May 1982, p. 54.
40. Brandt AM: Damaged goods: progressive medicine and social hygiene. In Brandt AM: *No Magic Bullet: A Social History of Venereal Disease in the United States since 1880.* Oxford University Press, New York, 1985, pp. 7–51.
41. Fee E and Krieger N: Understanding AIDS: historical interpretations and the limits of biomedical individualism. *Am J Public Health* 83: 1477–1486, 1993.
42. Centers for Disease Control and Prevention: Update: acquired immunodeficiency syndrome (AIDS)—United States. *Morb Mortal Wkly Rep* 32: 688–691, 1984.
43. Hearst N and Hulley SB: Preventing the heterosexual spread of AIDS: are we giving our patients the best advice? *JAMA* 259: 2428–2432, 1988.
44. Leviton LC: Theoretical foundations in AIDS-prevention programs. In Valdiserri RO (ed.): *Preventing AIDS: The Design of Effective Programs.* Rutgers University Press, New Brunswick, NJ, 1989, pp. 42–90.

45. Institute of Medicine: Summary and recommendations. In Institute of Medicine: *Confronting AIDS: Directions for Public Health, Health-care, and Research.* National Academy Press, Washington, DC, 1986, pp. 5–35.

46. Valdiserri RO, Janssen RJ, Buehler JW, and Fleming P: The context of HIV/AIDS surveillance. *J Acquir Immune Defic Syndr* 25: S97–S104, 2000.

47. Kaslow RA, Ostrow DG, Detels R, et al.: The Multicenter AIDS Cohort Study: rationale, organization, and selected characteristics of the participants. *Am J Epidemiol* 126: 310–318, 1987.

48. Polk BF, Fox R, Brookmeyer R, et al.: Predictors of the acquired immunodeficiency syndrome developing in a cohort of seropositive homosexual men. *N Engl J Med* 316: 61–66, 1987.

49. Valdiserri RO: HIV counseling and testing: its evolving role in HIV prevention. *AIDS Educ Prev* 9 (SB): 2–13, 1997.

50. U.S. Public Health Service: Coolfont report: a PHS plan for prevention and control of AIDS and the AIDS virus. *Public Health Rep* 101: 341–348, 1986.

51. Ambroziak J and Levy JA: Epidemiology, natural history, and pathogenesis of HIV infection. In Homles KK, Sparling PF, Mardh PA, Lemon SM, Stamm W, Piot P, and Wasserheit JN (eds.): *Sexually Transmitted Diseases*, 3rd ed. McGraw-Hill, New York, 1999, pp. 251–258.

52. Panem S: Lessons for the future. In Panem S: *The AIDS Bureaucracy: Why Society Failed to Meet the AIDS Crisis and How We Might Improve Our Response.* Harvard University Press, Cambridge, MA, 1988, pp. 136–149.

53. Panem S: Economics and politics. In Panem S: *The AIDS Bureaucracy: Why Society Failed to Meet the AIDS Crisis and How We Might Improve Our Response.* Harvard University Press, Cambridge, MA, 1988, pp. 72–85.

54. Allen SM, Mor V, Fleishman JA, and Piette JD: The organizational transformation of advocacy: growth and development of AIDS community-based organizations. *AIDS Public Policy* 10: 48–59, 1995.

55. Arno P: The nonprofit sector's response to the AIDS epidemic: community-based services in San Francisco. *Am J Public Health* 76: 1325–1330, 1986.

56. Valdiserri RO: Planning and implementing AIDS-prevention programs: a case study approach. In Valdiserri RO: *Preventing AIDS: The Design of Effective Programs.* Rutgers University Press, New Brunswick, NJ, 1989, pp. 1129–1208.

57. Freudenberg N, Lee J, and Silver D: How Black and Latino community organizations respond to the AIDS epidemic: a case study in one New York City neighborhood. *AIDS Educ Prev* 1: 12–21, 1989.

58. Wallace R: A synergism of plagues: "planned shrinkage," contagious housing destruction, and AIDS in the Bronx. *Environ Res* 47: 1–33, 1988.

59. Freudenberg N and Zimmerman MA: The role of community organizations in public health practice: the lessons from AIDS prevention. In: *AIDS Prevention in the Community.* American Public Health Association, Washington, DC, 1995, pp. 183–197.

60. Centers for Disease Control and Prevention: Changes in the public health system. *Morb Mortal Wkly Rep* 48: 1141–1147, 1999.

61. Bye LL, Henne JC, and Quarles RC: Designing an effective AIDS prevention campaign for San Francisco: results from the first probability sample of an urban gay male community. Paper presented at the International Conference on AIDS, Atlanta, GA, April 14–17, 1985.

62. Research and Decisions Corporation: *Designing an Effective AIDS Prevention Cam-*

paign Strategy for San Francisco: Results from the First Probability Sample of an Urban Gay Male Community. Research and Decisions Corporation, San Francisco, 1984, pp. 12–17.

63. Lyon E, Seibert J, and Dodds S: Risk reduction education package targeting gay and bisexual males: normative change through structured groups facilitated by trained non-professional volunteers. Paper presented at the International Conference on AIDS, Paris, June 23–25, 1986.

64. Samet RL, Christ GH, Dunne R, et al.: Tri-partite systems venture to meet the AIDS crisis in New York City. Paper presented at the International Conference on AIDS, Paris, June 23–25, 1986.

65. Hartgers C, van Ameijden EJC, van den Hoek JAR, and Coutinho RA: Needle sharing and participation in the Amsterdam syringe exchange program among HIV-seronegative injecting drug users. *Public Health Rep* 107: 675–681, 1992.

66. Anderson W: The New York needle trial: the politics of public health in the age of AIDS. In Berridge V and Strong P (eds.): *AIDS and Contemporary History.* Cambridge University Press, Cambridge, England, 1993, pp. 157–181.

67. Institute for Health Policy Studies: *The Public Health Impact of Needle Exchange Programs in the United States and Abroad: Summary, Conclusions, and Recommendations.* University of California, San Francisco, 1993, pp. 16–17.

68. Gostin L: The needle-borne HIV epidemic: causes and public health responses. *Behav Sci Law* 9: 287–304, 1991.

69. Elovich R, Sorge R: Toward a community-based needle exchange for New York City. *AIDS Public Policy* 6: 165–172, 1991.

70. Lambert B: Drug group to offer free needles to combat AIDS in New York City. *New York Times,* January 8, 1988, p. A-1.

71. Anderson W: The New York needle trial: the politics of public health in the age of AIDS. *Am J Public Health* 81: 1506–1517, 1991.

72. American Foundation for AIDS Research: AmFAR's decade of commitment to needle exchange. URL: www.amfar.org/decade, (1998).

73. Des Jarlais DC, Marmor M, Paone D, et al.: HIV incidence among injecting drug users in New York City syringe exchange programmes. *Lancet* 348: 987–991, 1996.

74. Lurie P and Drucker E: An opportunity lost: HIV infections associated with lack of a national needle-exchange programme in the USA. *Lancet* 349: 604–608, 1997.

75. Robins L and Backstrom C: Organizational imperatives and policy perspectives of AIDS community-based organizations: a view from the states. *AIDS Public Policy* 14: 3–19, 1999.

76. Kinsella J: The unphotogenic epidemic. In Kinsella J: *Covering the Plague: AIDS and the American Media.* Rutgers University Press, New Brunswick, NJ, 1989, pp. 122–145.

77. Thomas E: The new untouchables. *Time,* September 23, 1985, pp. 24–26.

78. Herreck GM: AIDS and stigma. *Am Behav Sci* 42: 1106–1116, 1999.

79. Centers for Disease Control and Prevention: Provisional Public Health Service inter-agency recommendations for screening donated blood and plasma for antibody to the virus causing acquired immunodeficiency syndrome. *Morb Mortal Wkly Rep* 34: 1–5, 1985.

80. Centers for Disease Control and Prevention: Update: Public Health Service workshop on human T-lymphotropic virus type III antibody testing—United States. *Morb Mortal Wkly Rep* 34: 477–478, 1985.

81. Centers for Disease Control and Prevention: Revision of the case definition of Ac-

quired Immunodeficiency Syndrome for national reporting—United States. *Morb Mortal Wkly Rep* 34: 373–375, 1985.

82. Centers for Disease Control and Prevention: Recommendations for assisting in the prevention of perinatal transmission of human T-lymphotropic virus type III/lymphadenopathy-associated virus and the acquired immunodeficiency syndrome. *Morb Mortal Wkly Rep* 34: 721–726 and 731–732, 1985.

83. National Institutes of Health: The impact of routine HTLV-III antibody testing on public health. Paper presented at the Consensus Development Conference, Bethesda, MD, July 7–9, 1986.

84. Brook I: Approval of zidovudine (AZT) for acquired immunodeficiency syndrome: a challenge to the medial and pharmaceutical communities. *JAMA* 258: 1517, 1987.

85. National Gay Rights Advocates: *AIDS and Your Legal Rights.* San Francisco: National Gay Rights Advocates, 1986.

86. Lyter DW, Valdiserri RO, Kingsley LA, Amoroso WP, and Rinaldo CR: The HIV antibody test: why gay and bisexual men want or do not want to know their results. *Public Health Rep* 102: 468–474, 1987.

87. Brandt AM: The syphilis epidemic and its relation to AIDS. *Science* 239: 375–380, 1988.

88. Brandt AM: AIDS: from social history to social policy. In Fee E and Fox DM (eds.): *AIDS: The Burdens of History.* University of California Press, Berkeley, 1988, pp. 147–171.

89. Brandt AM: AIDS in historical perspective: four lessons from the history of sexually transmitted diseases. *Am J Public Health* 78: 367–371, 1988.

90. Bayer R, Levine C, and Wolf SM: HIV antibody screening: an ethical framework for evaluating proposed programs. *JAMA* 256: 1768–1774, 1986.

91. Institute of Medicine: Opportunities for altering the course of the epidemic. In Institute of Medicine: *Confronting AIDS: Directions for Public Health, Health-Care, and Research.* National Academy Press, Washington, DC, 1986, pp. 95–137.

92. Hunter N: AIDS prevention and civil liberties: the false security of mandatory testing. *SIECUS Rep* 16: 1–9, 1987.

93. Centers for Disease Control and Prevention: Testing donors of organs, tissues, and semen for antibody to human T-lymphotropic virus type III/lymphadenopathy-associated virus. *Morb Mortal Wkly Rep* 34: 294, 1985.

94. Centers for Disease Control and Prevention: Additional recommendations to reduce sexual and drug abuse–related transmission of human T-lymphotropic virus type III/lymphadenopathy-associated virus. *Morb Mortal Wkly Rep* 35: 152–155, 1986.

95. Friedland GH and Klein RS: Transmission of the human immunodeficiency virus. *N Engl J Med* 317: 1125–1135, 1987.

96. Friedland GH, Saltzman BR, Rogers MF, Kahl PA, Lesser ML, Mayers MM, and Klein RS: Lack of transmission of HTLV-III/LAV infection to household contacts of patients with AIDS or AIDS-related complex with oral candidiasis. *N Engl J Med* 314: 344–349, 1986.

97. Berthier A, Fauchet R, Genetet N, Pommereuil M, Chamaret S, Fonlupt J, et al.: Transmissibility of human immunodeficiency virus in haemophilic and non-haemophilic children living in a private school in France. *Lancet* ii (8507): 598–601, 1986.

98. Centers for Disease Control and Prevention: Recommendations for preventing transmission of infection with human T-lymphotropic virus type III/lymphadenopathy-associated virus in the workplace. *Morb Mortal Wkly Rep* 34: 681–686 and 691–695, 1985.

99. Centers for Disease Control and Prevention: Education and foster care of children infected with human T-lymphotropic virus type III/lymphadenopathy-associated virus. *Morb Mortal Wkly Rep* 34: 517–521, 1985.

100. Gostin L: The AIDS Litigation Project: a national review of court and Human Rights Commission decisions, part II: discrimination. *JAMA* 263: 2086–2093, 1990.

101. Valdiserri RO: Epidemics in perspective. *J Med Hum Bioethics* 8: 95–100, 1987.

102. Presidential Commission on the Human Immunodeficiency Virus Epidemic: Legal and ethical issues. In Presidential Commission on the Human Immunodeficiency Virus Epidemic: *Report of the Presidential Commission on the Human Immunodeficiency Virus Epidemic.* U.S. Government Printing Office, Washington, DC, 1988, pp. 119–140.

103. World Health Organization Global Programme on AIDS: *Avoidance of Discrimination in Relation to HIV Infected People and People with AIDS* (WHA41.24). World Health Organization, Geneva, 1988.

104. Annas GJ: Protecting patients from discrimination: the Americans with Disabilities Act and HIV infection. *N Engl J Med* 339: 1255–1259, 1998.

105. Gostin LA, Feldblum C, and Webber DW: Disability discrimination in America: HIV/AIDS and other health conditions. *JAMA* 281: 745–752, 1999.

106. Office of the United Nations High Commissioner for Human Rights and the Joint United Nations Programme on HIV/AIDS: *HIV/AIDS and Human Rights International Guidelines (HR/PUB/98/1). United Nations, Geneva, 1998.*

107. Lee PR and Arno PS: AIDS and health policy. In Griggs J (ed.): *AIDS Public Policy Dimensions.* United Hospital Fund of New York, New York, 1987, pp. 3–20.

108. Osborn JE: AIDS: the challenge to ambulatory care. *J Ambulatory Care Manage* 11: 19–26, 1988.

109. Silverman M: AIDS care: the San Francisco model. *J Ambulatory Care Manag* 11: 14–18, 1988.

110. Howell EM: The role of community-based organizations in responding to the AIDS epidemic: examples from the HRSA Service Demonstrations. *J Public Health Policy* 12: 165–174, 1991.

111. Rosenblum LS, Buehler, JW, Morgan M, and Moien M: Increasing impact of HIV infection on hospitalizations in the United States, 1983–1988. *J Acquir Immune Defic Syndr* 5: 497–504, 1992.

112. Andrulis DP, Weslowski VB, and Gage LS: The 1987 U.S. hospital AIDS survey. *JAMA* 262: 784–794, 1989.

113. World Bank: Coping with the impact of HIV/AIDS. In World Bank: *Confronting AIDS: Public Priorities in a Global Epidemic.* Oxford University Press, Oxford, 1997, pp. 173–237.

114. Shulman LC and Mantell JE: The AIDS crisis: a United States health-care perspective. *Soc Sci Med* 26: 979–988, 1988.

115. Andriote JM: Advance and retreat. In Andriote JM: *Victory Deferred: How AIDS Changed Gay Life in America.* University of Chicago Press, Chicago, 1999, pp. 211–256.

116. United States Conference of Mayors: Landmark Ryan White CARE Act enacted. *AIDS Info Exchange* 7: 1–6, 1990.

117. Marx R, Katz MH, Park MS, and Gurley RJ: Meeting the service needs of HIV-infected persons: is the Ryan White CARE Act succeeding? *J Acquir Immune Defic Syndr* 14: 44–55, 1997.

118. Levi J and Kates J: HIV: challenging the health-care delivery system. *Am J Public Health* 90: 1033–1036, 2000.

119. Kaiser Family Foundation: *Financing HIV/AIDS Care: A Quilt with Many Holes* (pub. no. 1607), Henry J. Kaiser Family Foundation, Washington DC, 2000.

120. Joint United Nations Programme on HIV/AIDS: *Access to Drugs.* United Nations, Geneva, 1998.

121. Joint United Nations Programme on HIV/AIDS: Towards the creation of strategic partnerships: improving access to drugs for HIV/AIDS (98.40). United Nations, Geneva, 1998.

122. Rosenberg T: How to solve the world's AIDS crisis. *NY Times Magazine*, January 28, 2001, pp. 26–31, 52, 58, 62–63.

123. Brugha R and Walt G: A global health fund: a leap of faith? *Br Med J* 323: 152–154, 2001.

124. Tomes N: The making of a germ panic, then and now. *Am J Public Health* 90: 191–198, 2000.

125. Fischl MA, Richman DD, Grieco MH, Gottlieb MS, Volberding PA, Laskin OL, et al.: The efficacy of azidothymidine (AZT) in the treatment of patients with AIDS and AIDS-related complex. *N Engl J Med* 317: 185–191, 1987.

126. Volberding PA, Lagakos SW, Koch MA, Pettinelli C, Myers MW, Booth DK, et al.: Zidovudine in asymptomatic human immunodeficiency virus infection. *N Engl J Med* 322: 941–949, 1990.

127. Fischl MA, Richman DD, Hansen N, Collier AC, Carey JT, Para MF, et al.: The safety and efficacy of zidovudine (AZT) in the treatment of patients with mildly symptomatic HIV infection: a double blind, placebo-controlled trial. *Ann Intern Med* 112: 727–737, 1990.

128. Centers for Disease Control and Prevention: Zidovudine for the prevention of HIV transmission from mother to infant. *Morb Mortal Wkly Rep* 43: 285–287, 1994.

129. Connor EM, Sperling RS, Gelber R, Kiselev P, Scott G, O'Sullivan MJ, et al.: Reduction of maternal–infant transmission of human immunodeficiency virus type 1 with zidovudine treatment. *N Engl J Med* 331: 1173–1180, 1994.

130. Concorde Coordinating Committee: Concorde: MRC/ANRS randomised double-blind controlled trial of immediate and deferred zidovudine in symptom-free HIV infection. *Lancet* 343: 871–881, 1994.

131. Staszewski S, Loveday C, Picazo JJ, Dellamonica P, Skinhojm P, Johnson MA, et al.: Safety and efficacy of lamivudine–zidovudine combination therapy in zidovudine-experienced patients: a randomized controlled comparison with zidovudine monotherapy. *JAMA* 276: 111–117, 1996.

132. Katlama C, Ingrand D, Loveday C, Clumeck N, Mallolas J, Staszewski S, et al.: Safety and efficacy of lamivudine–zidovudine combination therapy in antiretroviral-naive patients: a randomized controlled comparison with zidovudine monotherapy. *JAMA* 276: 118–125, 1996.

133. Hammer SM, Katzenstein DA, Hughes MD, Gundacker H, Schooley RT, Haubrich RH, et al.: A trial comparing nucleoside monotherapy with combination therapy in HIV-infected adults with CD4 cell counts from 200 to 500 per cubic millimeter. *N Engl J Med* 335: 1081–1090, 1996.

134. Deeks SG, Smith M, Holodniy M, and Kahn JO: HIV-1 protease inhibitors: a review for clinicians. *JAMA* 277: 145–153, 1997.

135. Collier AC, Coombs RW, Schoenfeld DA, Bassett RL, Timpone J, Baruch A, et al.: Treatment of human immunodeficiency virus infection with saquinavir, zidovudine, and zalcitabine. *N Engl J Med* 334: 1011–1017, 1996.

136. Centers for Disease Control and Prevention: Update: trends in AIDS incidence, deaths, and prevalence—United States, 1996. *Morb Mortal Wkly Rep* 46: 165–173, 1997.

137. Palella FJ, Delaney KM, Moorman AC, Loveless MO, Fuhrer J, Satten GA, et al.: Declining morbidity and mortality among patients with advanced human immuno-deficiency virus infection. *N Engl J Med* 338: 853–860, 1998.

138. CASCADE Collaboration: Survival after introduction of HAART in people with known duration of HIV-1 infection. *Lancet* 355: 1158–1159, 2000.

139. Sullivan A: When plagues end. *New York Times*, November 10, 1996, pp. 6, 52.

140. Carr A and Cooper DA: Adverse effects of antiretroviral therapy. *Lancet* 356: 1423–1430, 2000.

141. Furtado MR, Callaway DS, Phair JP, Kunstman KJ, Stanton JL, Macken CA, Perelson AS, and Wolinsky SM: Persistence of HIV-1 transcription in peripheral-blood mononuclear cells in patients receiving potent antiretroviral therapy. *N Engl J Med* 340: 1614–1622, 1999.

142. Centers for Disease Control and Prevention: *HIV/AIDS Surveillance Report* 12: 1–44, 2000.

143. Kaiser Family Foundation: *HIV/AIDS Research: Successes Bring New Challenges.* Henry J. Kaiser Family Foundation, Washington DC, 2000.

144. Office of Technology Assessment: *How Has Federal Research on AIDS/HIV Disease Contributed to Other Fields?* Office of Technology Assessment, Washington, DC, 1990.

145. Wachter RM: AIDS, activism, and the politics of health. *N Engl J Med* 326: 128–132, 1992.

146. Valdiserri RO, Tama GM, and Ho M: The role of community advisory committees in clinical trials of anti-HIV agents. *IRB: Rev Hum Subj Res* 10: 5–7, 1988.

147. McGuire J: Inclusion, representation, and parity: the making of a public health response to HIV. In Mayer KH and Pizer HF (eds.): *The Emergence of AIDS: The Impact on Immunology, Microbiology, and Public Health.* American Public Health Association, Washington, DC, 2000, pp. 181–205.

148. Edgar H and Rothman DJ: New rules for new drugs: the challenge of AIDS to the regulatory process. *Millbank Quart* 68: 111–142, 1990.

149. Valdiserri RO, Aultman TV, and Curran JW: Community planning: a national strategy to improve HIV prevention programs. *J Community Health* 20: 87–100, 1995.

150. Bowen GS, Marconi K, Kohn S, Bailey DM, Goosby EP, Shorter S, and Niemcryk S: First year of AIDS services delivery under title I of the Ryan White CARE Act. *Public Health Rep* 107: 491–499, 1992.

151. Office of AIDS Research, National Institutes of Health: OAR Advisory Council. URL: www.nih.gov/od/oar/about/oarac (October 2000).

152. Kushner T: *Angels in America. Part 2: Perestroika.* Theatre Communications Group, New York, 1992, p. 148.

153. Ziegler P: *The Black Death.* Harper and Row, New York, 1969, p. 45.

154. National Institute of Allergy and Infectious Diseases: HIV vaccine development status report. URL: www.niaid.nih.gov/daids/vaccine (May 2000).

155. Holtgrave DR, Qualls NL, Curran JW, Valdiserri RO, Guinan ME, and Parra WC: An overview of the effectiveness and efficiency of HIV prevention programs. *Public Health Rep* 110: 134–146, 1995.

156. National Institutes of Health: Interventions to prevent HIV risk behaviors. *NIH Consensus Statement* 15: 1–41, February 11–13, 1997.

Appendix
HIV/AIDS: Chronology of an Unfolding Epidemic

June 5, 1981:	*Morbidity and Mortality Weekly Report,* report of *Pneumocystis* pneumonia
1982:	San Francisco AIDS Foundation incorporated
1982:	Gay Men's Health Crisis founded in New York City
July 1982:	New syndrome is named AIDS (acquired immune deficiency syndrome) by researchers and U.S. government officials
1983:	National Association of People with AIDS (NAPWA) formed
February 1983:	National AIDS Hotline established by U.S. federal government
March 1983:	U.S. Government issues first guidelines on the prevention of AIDS
May 1983:	French isolate T-lymphotropic retrovirus (LAV) from patient at risk for AIDS
May 25, 1983:	Assistant U.S. Secretary of Health, Edward Brandt, labels AIDS the nation's "number one health priority" in a front-page story in the *New York Times*
July 1983:	San Francisco General Hospital opens an AIDS ward
1984:	Americans isolate T-lymphotropic retrovirus (HTLV-III) from patients with or at risk for AIDS
1984:	CDC funds the U.S. Conference of Mayors to provide seed funding and technical assistance to CBOs for AIDS-prevention efforts
1984:	Numerous serologic studies demonstrate antibodies to HTLV-III/LAV among persons with or at risk for AIDS
1984:	Syringe exchange program implemented in Amsterdam to reduce HIV and HBV transmission among IDUs
April 1984:	NIH funded longitudinal study of the natural history of AIDS in Baltimore, Chicago, Los Angeles, and Pittsburgh (Multicenter AIDS Cohort Study: MACS)
July 15, 1984:	WHO reports 421 AIDS cases in Europe (Denmark, France, Germany, Greece, Italy, Netherlands, Spain, Sweden, Switzerland, United Kingdom)
1985:	American Foundation for AIDS Research (AmFAR) is founded
January 1985:	U.S. Public Health Service publishes provisional recommendations on the screening of donated blood/plasma for HTLV-III/LAV
March 1985:	FDA licenses assay to screen donated blood for antibodies to HTLV-III
April 1985:	CDC provides funding to health departments for "alternate test sites"
April 1985:	First International Conference on AIDS, Atlanta
July 1985:	*Life* magazine cover story: "No One Is Safe from AIDS" helps make AIDS a heterosexual concern
July 25, 1985:	Public announcement that Rock Hudson has AIDS

September 1985:	Indiana teenager Ryan White, a hemophiliac with AIDS, is refused entry into school
Fall 1985:	U.S. Public Health Service Executive Task Force on AIDS calls for elimination of HTLV-III/LAV infection by 2000
October 1985:	U.S. Department of Defense begins routine testing of military applicants for HTLV-III/LAV
October 2, 1985:	American film star Rock Hudson dies of AIDS
January 1986:	CDC announces funding to health-departments for AIDS health education and risk-reduction efforts
February 1986:	*Morbidity and Mortality Weekly Report* reports "suspicion" that HTLV-III/LAV infection may be responsible for increased tuberculosis morbidity
March 1986:	CDC issues recommendations encouraging testing and counseling among high-risk groups
May 1986:	The virus's name is changed to "human immunodeficiency virus" at the suggestion of an international scientific panel
June 1986:	National network of AIDS clinical research units is established by the NIH (AIDS Clinical Trial Groups)
June 4, 1986:	U.S. Public Health Service meets at Coolfont, West Virginia, to plan AIDS strategy
October 1986:	Institute of Medicine and National Academy of Sciences issue "Confronting AIDS," which recommends a major educational campaign, voluntary testing, trials to provide easier access to sterile syringes for IDUs, and systems of community-based care for persons with AIDS
October 1986:	CDC reports that cumulative incidences of AIDS among blacks and Hispanics are three times that of whites
October 1986:	Surgeon General Koop releases his "Report on Acquired Immune Deficiency," calling for AIDS education "at the earliest grade possible"
1987:	"And the Band Played On," in which Randy Shilts detailed the history of the early days of AIDS in America, is published
1987:	State and local departments of education begin to collect information from high school students on HIV-related knowledge, beliefs, and behaviors
February 1987:	World Health Organization launches its Global Programme on AIDS
March 1987:	AIDS Coalition to Unleash Power (ACT UP) formed in New York City by playwright and activist Larry Kramer
March 19, 1987:	FDA approves AZT—the first specific antiretroviral treatment
June 8, 1987:	In response to a congressional directive, Public Health Service adds HIV infection to the list of "dangerous contagious diseases" for which aliens can be excluded from the United States
August 1987:	First U.S. clinical trial of an HIV vaccine in humans conducted at the National Institutes of Health

August 1987:	CDC recommends that blood and body fluid precautions be used for all patients, regardless of serostatus ("universal precautions")
October 11, 1987:	AIDS Memorial Quilt first displayed on the Washington Mall
1988:	Application of the PCR (polymerase chain reaction) test to diagnosis of HIV
January 1, 1988:	HIV replaces HTLV-III/LAV in the International Classification of Diseases codes
May 1988:	CDC announces direct prevention funding to racial and ethnic minority national organizations
May–June 1988:	Surgeon General Koop mails "Understanding AIDS" to every American household
June 1988:	Report of the first Presidential Commission on the HIV Epidemic, calling for HIV prevention education, early diagnosis of HIV infection, stronger privacy protection for persons with HIV, and improved capacity to treat substance abuse
October 11, 1988:	Protesters shut down the FDA, demanding a quicker approval process for AIDS treatment
November 1988:	New York City Health Department begins the Needle Exchange Pilot Program, the first government-funded needle-exchange program in the United States
November 1988:	NIH Office of AIDS Research established
December 1, 1988:	Institution of annual World AIDS Day by the World Health Organization Global Programme on AIDS
December 20, 1988:	Max Robinson, former ABC news anchor and nationally prominent black journalist, dies of AIDS
1989:	United Nations Centre for Human Rights and World Health Organization Global Programme on AIDS hold first international consultation on AIDS and human rights
1989:	Based on congressional mandate, CDC begins direct funding of CBOs
July 1989:	100,000 cases of AIDS reported in the United States
1990:	Americans with Disabilities Act enacted (AIDS identified as a disability)
1990:	FDA announces expanded availability of investigational new HIV/AIDS drugs through a parallel-track mechanism
July 1990:	CDC reports on possible transmission of HIV to a patient during an invasive dental procedure
August 1990:	Ryan White Comprehensive AIDS Resources Emergency (CARE) Act signed into law by President George H.W. Bush
1991:	FOX becomes the first broadcast network to air a condom ad at the national level
July 1991:	CDC issues guidelines on the prevention of HIV and hepatitis B (HBV) to patients during "exposure-prone" invasive procedures
November 1991:	Basketball star Earvin "Magic" Johnson announces his HIV infection
April 8, 1992:	Tennis star Arthur Ashe announces that he has AIDS

1993:	AIDS becomes the leading cause of death among 25–44-year-old Americans
March 1993:	U.S. Government Accounting Office (GAO) reports that needle-exchange programs "may hold some promise" as an AIDS prevention strategy
1994:	European "Concorde" study shows no significant clinical or survival benefit from the early use of ZDV (zidovudine) in asymptomatic persons
February 24, 1994:	NIH announces effectiveness of ZDV (zidovudine) in preventing perinatal transmission
1995:	Joint United Nations Programme on HIV/AIDS (UNAIDS) established
1995:	Olympic gold medalist Greg Louganis announces he is HIV positive
May 1995:	Identification of the viral cause of Kaposi's sarcoma (HHV-8)
December 1995:	FDA approves the first protease inhibitor (saquinavir)
1996:	Home-collection HIV testing approved by the FDA
1996:	Substantial declines reported in U.S. AIDS deaths and incidence of opportunistic infections—related to improvements in early diagnosis and treatment
September 1996:	International Guidelines on HIV/AIDS and Human Rights produced by U.N. High Commissioner for Human Rights and the U.N. Programme on HIV/AIDS
February 18, 1997:	DHHS secretary's report to Labor/HHS Committee on Appropriations, finding that "needle exchange programs can be an effective component of a comprehensive strategy to prevent HIV"
1998:	U.S. Supreme Court rules that Americans with Disabilities Act covers those in early stages of HIV disease (*Bragdon v. Abbott*)
March 1998:	National Black Leadership Commission on AIDS declares that the HIV/AIDS epidemic has reached a "state of emergency" in African American and other minority communities
June 1998:	VaxGen begins first phase III (efficacy) trial of an HIV vaccine, based on GP120 protein
July 1998:	Case report of sexual transmission of an HIV-1 strain resistant to multiple reverse-transcriptase and protease inhibitors
March 1998:	Short-course ZDV (zidovudine) shown effective in reducing the risk of perinatal HIV transmission
October 1999:	U.S. Congress provides $100 million increase in U.S. support to sub-Saharan Africa and India to strengthen HIV prevention and care efforts ("LIFE" initiative)
June 2000:	United Nations Security Council discusses HIV/AIDS as a "threat" to international security
July 2000:	Researchers at the Thirteenth International AIDS Conference in Durban, South Africa, report that nonoxynol-9 (N-9) does not protect against HIV transmission and may have caused more transmission among women who used the microbicide

July 2000:	Call for a global fund to support HIV/AIDS, TB, and malaria, at the G8 Summit, Okinawa, Japan
March 2001:	Several drug manufacturers (Bristol-Myers Squibb, Merck, and Abbott Laboratories) agree to reduce cost of AIDS drugs in Africa and other developing countries
June 1, 2001:	CDC releases a study showing high rates of new HIV infection among young men who have sex with men (MSM) in 7 U.S. cities, suggesting a possible resurgence of HIV
June 25–27, 2001:	United National General Assembly holds a special session on HIV/AIDS calling for enhanced coordination and intensification of national, regional, and international efforts to combat the epidemic in a comprehensive manner
April 2002:	Global Fund to Fight AIDS, TB, and Malaria makes its first round of grants

2

HIV and AIDS Surveillance: Public Health Lessons Learned

JAMES W. BUEHLER

To prevent and control specific diseases, public health has an ongoing need to monitor trends in the occurrence and characteristics of particular health problems. This process is called "public health surveillance," and the structures and procedures used to conduct this monitoring are called "surveillance systems." Typically, surveillance efforts grow from ad hoc systems developed in response to the recognition of new problems to more elaborate systems that evolve as prevention and control programs are established (1). This is indeed the case with surveillance systems aimed at monitoring the epidemic of human immunodeficiency virus (HIV) and acquired immunodeficiency syndrome (AIDS). HIV/AIDS surveillance has included not only monitoring the various stages of HIV infection and associated diseases, including AIDS, but also monitoring the behaviors that place individuals at risk for infection, as well as the use of preventive or treatment services by those at risk for, or already infected with, HIV.

Surveillance systems are called on to address a range of questions that can be distilled into the four basic parameters of when, where, who, and what (1). For HIV, these questions include the following:

When: What are the temporal trends in HIV infections, associated diseases including AIDS, and health-related behaviors that affect the risk or outcome of HIV infection?

Where: Where are HIV infections occurring, and where are the populations at greatest risk for infection located?

Who: Who is being affected by the epidemic?

What: What are the clinical manifestations and outcomes of HIV infection? What is the nature or properties of the HIV virus itself (e.g., what are the predominant strains, what are the emerging patterns of antiretroviral resistance)?

To assess their ability to answer these questions, we can judge surveillance systems by multiple measures (2): What is their level of simplicity or complexity? How flexible are they in responding to changing circumstances or information needs? What is the quality of the information that is obtained? How acceptable are reporting procedures to those whose ongoing support is required for maintaining surveillance? What is their ability to detect all events of interest or a representative sample of such events? How timely are reports in providing information to the array of potential users? What is their "predictive value" in assuring that reported events are indeed measuring the intended outcome? How stable or consistent are systems in ensuring that observed trends represent true trends rather than reporting artifacts? A brief reflection on these diverse measures will yield the conclusion that individual surveillance attributes can often be at odds with one another. For example, pressures to increase the timeliness of reporting may lead to decreased completeness or data quality. Thus, the success of any surveillance system depends on how well these competing attributes are balanced to meet priority public health needs.

This chapter considers some of the important lessons learned from HIV/AIDS surveillance during the first two decades of the epidemic. Public health's experience with HIV/AIDS has drawn surveillance from the background into the forefront, and a detailed discussion of these lessons will show their increasing relevance to the broader domain of public health practice.

Background

As with many diseases, the manifestations of HIV infection were first recognized in their most severe or dramatic form, the constellation of diseases known as "AIDS" (3,4). Consequently, surveillance initially focused on AIDS, and even at the time of this writing AIDS reporting remains the only form of HIV-related surveillance that is conducted by every U.S. state and territory (as of 2002, thirty-five states or territories required HIV reporting by name (5). Initially, AIDS surveillance was primarily an indicator of population groups at greatest risk for HIV infection. More recently, as a result of advances in care, AIDS surveillance data are likely to represent those who have not benefited from early diagnosis and care of HIV infection or those for whom new treatments have ceased to be effective (4).

Perhaps the greatest challenge for HIV/AIDS surveillance has been the need to rapidly adapt to changing information needs. During the course of the epidemic, HIV/AIDS surveillance systems have had to respond to a succession of major events, developments, and advances, including the discovery of HIV, the burgeoning recognition of the broad and diverse spectrum of HIV-related disease, the characterization of the role of progressive immune deficiency as the underlying disease mechanism, shifts in population groups most affected by the epidemic, recognition of different strains of the virus, dramatic advances in clinical evaluation and treatment, and significant alterations in the course of the disease as the result of highly active antiretroviral therapies.

Throughout its course, the HIV/AIDS epidemic has drawn unprecedented attention to the process and practice of public health surveillance, a previously unheralded dimension of public health. There are multiple reasons for this attention, shaped by the public health and social impacts of the epidemic, including the responses of government agencies and advocacy groups. One reason that surveillance systems for HIV/AIDS have been scrutinized is because they serve as the basis for allocation of federal program funds for both prevention and care, most notably funding to states and large cities from the Centers for Disease Control and Prevention (CDC) for HIV prevention programs (6) and from the Health Resources and Services Administration (HRSA) for programs supported under the Ryan White Care Act (7). Thus, criteria developed for purposes of public health surveillance—for example, the surveillance case definition for AIDS— have been called on to serve other purposes. Another example is the use of the AIDS case definition to determine eligibility for benefits from the Social Security Administration (8,9). Other factors contributing to this increased focus on HIV/AIDS surveillance include the substantial investment of public funds to support these efforts and heightened concerns about the privacy and confidentiality of HIV/AIDS surveillance systems, as typified by the long-standing and ongoing debate since 1986 over whether HIV infection should be reportable by name to health departments (10,11).

Ironically, and despite the tremendous efforts that have been invested in HIV/AIDS surveillance, the most important questions have remained largely elusive: How many new HIV infections are occurring each year in the United States (i.e., what is the HIV incidence)? Who are those becoming newly infected? Among those at highest risk for HIV infection, what are the trends in behaviors that can lead to exposure to HIV? There are multiple reasons for difficulties in answering these questions. Regarding the assessment of HIV incidence, new HIV infections are often not recognized or diagnosed, and the early stages of infection may be asymptomatic for years. Thus, detection of infections depends on the use of HIV testing. Until recently, it has not been possible to determine who among those newly diagnosed with HIV were newly infected (12), and the large-scale use of special tests to determine trends in recent infections in the U.S. will not go into effect until 2003–2004. As a result, diagnosed infections represent an unknown percentage of newly occurring infections, although efforts to improve measures of HIV incidence are the focus of ongoing research.

Before the advent of highly active antiretroviral therapy, it was possible to estimate HIV incidence by combining information on trends in the number of persons reported with AIDS with information on the reasonably well-characterized time from infection to development of AIDS (13). This mathematical technique asked and answered the question, What are the numbers of HIV infections that must have occurred to give rise to observed cases of AIDS? However, this "back-calculation" method has been rendered obsolete by successes in treatment, which have removed a critical factor (knowledge about the time from infection to the development of AIDS) from the equation (14).

Regarding monitoring of behaviors associated with risk of HIV infection, these, too, are difficult to track—because they are very private behaviors (e.g., sexual practices, illicit drug use). Additionally, populations at highest risk for HIV are often stigmatized, either implicitly by prevalent social norms or attitudes (e.g., attitudes regarding homosexuality and drug use, racism) or explicitly by laws and regulations (e.g., sodomy laws, criminalization of sexual and drug-using of behaviors associated with HIV transmission) (15,16). Together, these effects complicate the measurement in risk behavior trends, particularly among those groups who are most vulnerable or susceptible to becoming infected with HIV.

Against this backdrop, some of the lessons learned from HIV/AIDS surveillance can now be addressed.

Lesson 1: Multiple Surveillance Methods for Monitoring Complicated Diseases

Surveillance methods tend to fall somewhere along a spectrum defined by the following polarity: it is possible to collect a relatively limited amount of information about a large number of people, or it is possible to collect more detailed information about a smaller number of people. This polarity can be illustrated by considering an analyst working with a large, national computer file of HIV-related death certificates compared with an ethnographer who spends an extended period observing behaviors among a few subjects at risk for HIV infection. Both can yield important insights into the HIV epidemic—the former by providing a broad population-level overview, and the latter by providing clues to the more individual and personal behaviors that shape the course of the epidemic. Not surprisingly, the answers provided by AIDS surveillance (collecting a little information about many) raised new questions, which required alternative surveillance approaches.

This first became apparent as "alternative" (i.e., to routine notifiable disease reporting) data sources and methods were used to assess the completeness of

AIDS reporting (17) and to describe the broader spectrum of severe HIV-related disease that was not captured by AIDS reporting criteria (18,19), This led to an expanded use of hospital discharge data and vital statistics as an adjunct to AIDS reporting, not only to describe the full spectrum of HIV-related morbidity and mortality but also to provide a "backstop" to ensure more complete reporting of AIDS cases (20,21). This also led to the development of supplemental surveillance systems, whereby a subset of states obtained more in-depth information on both the pediatric and adult spectrum of HIV-related disease (22,23). These supplemental surveillance projects were initiated in a limited number of states, rather than all states, because they required more effort and expertise to manage and coordinate than routine case reporting.

The need for more detailed information on risk behaviors and the use of preventive and other health services led to development of the Supplement to HIV/AIDS Surveillance Project (24). This project, also conducted in a limited number of states, expanded routine HIV/AIDS case-reporting procedures to include more in-depth interviews of persons reported with HIV/AIDS. Categories of information collection included an expanded (compared with the routine HIV/AIDS report forms) demographic profile, HIV risk behavior information, access to and use of health services, and (for women) reproductive history. The HIV Testing Survey (HITS) is another example of a supplemental surveillance system (25). The HITS survey is intended to assess risk behaviors and the use of HIV testing services among selected groups, in part to assess the representativeness of HIV reports. A number of other surveys, while not exclusively developed to monitor the HIV epidemic, have been used to monitor the use of HIV testing and relevant behaviors (e.g., condom use) among the "general population." These include the Youth Risk Behavioral Surveillance System, which targets adolescents, the Behavioral Risk Factor Surveillance System, a general-population telephone survey conducted by states, the National Survey of Family Growth, and the National Health Interview Survey (26,27).

Following the discovery of HIV, two separate lines of surveillance evolved to monitor HIV infection itself: HIV infection reporting using the notifiable disease approach (28) and the institution of a "family" of HIV seroprevalence surveys among an array of U.S. populations with varying levels of HIV risk (29,30,31). These included "unlinked" seroprevalence surveys (e.g., surveys in which identifying information is removed from specimens before HIV testing, rendering them anonymous), as well as HIV prevalence data from other agencies that conduct routine screening, including data on first-time blood donors, military recruits, and applicants to the Jobs Corps, a residential training program for disadvantaged youth. The unlinked HIV seroprevalence surveys were based on testing "leftover" blood that had been routinely collected for other purposes (e.g., syphilis testing) and would otherwise have been discarded. Before testing, all personally identifying information was removed from the specimens. With the exception of the Survey of Childbearing Women, which was based on detecting maternal HIV antibodies in blood left over from newborn metabolic screening, these unlinked surveys were conducted in settings where voluntary HIV counseling and testing was routinely available to those clients who wanted to know their HIV status, such as drug treatment centers and clinics for sexually transmitted disease.

Over time, the unlinked HIV seroprevalence surveys have been phased out in the United States. This occurred because the epidemiologic utility of the clinic-based surveys waned as trends stabilized and the surveys began to yield fewer new insights; because controversies regarding the ethics of unlinked testing were renewed as new treatments became available; and because the resulting political liabilities associated with these controversies, particularly for the Survey of Childbearing Women (32) became too great to justify continued support for this approach to HIV surveillance in the United States. As a result, the network of unlinked seroprevalence surveys has been replaced by a more focused group of studies aimed at estimating HIV incidence using the so-called "detuned" HIV assay, a testing strategy which can detect recent HIV infections (12,33).

Although assessing disease prevalence and incidence is generally considered a public health surveillance function, it is also possible to develop estimates by using data aggregated from research studies, which may have been time-limited and not part of an ongoing surveillance system. An example of this approach is the assessment of HIV incidence among drug injectors in New York City, based on an analysis of ten studies employing three broad types of methods (cohort studies, studies of injection drug users who accepted voluntary HIV testing during successive visits to a needle exchange program or a sexually transmitted disease clinic, and studies of persons who accepted voluntary counseling and testing at a drug treatment center) (34). Another example is the expert consensus process used by the San Francisco Department of Public Health to estimate HIV incidence trends in the city by using multiple data sources, including clinic records, data from voluntary counseling and testing services, and various research studies (35).

Thus, an array of surveillance methods have been developed, ranging from notifiable disease reporting of HIV and AIDS cases, which involve collection of a relatively limited amount of information about all persons reported with AIDS (all states) or HIV infection (an increasing number of states), to the aggregate analyses of data from studies or projects that in themselves may not be considered surveillance systems. If the full epidemiologic picture of the epidemic is considered to be a mosaic, the approach of employing multiple surveillance methods attempts to provide as many of the tiles as possible to describe key trends in the epidemic, knowing that certain critical pieces of information are either unavailable or very difficult to obtain for a mix of reasons.

The multiphased continuum from HIV risk to infection and disease, along with the array of surveillance methods that have been called on to address the HIV epidemic, highlight the importance of using a combination of surveillance methods for complex public health problems. While a multifaceted approach to surveillance is not unique to HIV/AIDS, the resources available in the United States to implement HIV/AIDS surveillance have allowed for the development of this approach to an unprecedented level. One example of the positive legacy of public health's experience with these expanded surveillance approaches can be seen in the U.S. plan for monitoring emerging infectious diseases (36).

Lesson 2: Behavioral Surveillance a Critical Adjunct to "General Population" Surveys

Behavioral data from a number of sources have informed HIV/AIDS-related public health efforts. For example, the National Survey of Family Growth has monitored trends in sexual behaviors and contraceptive use among women (37). The AIDS supplement of the National Health Interview Survey has provided data on HIV-related knowledge and attitudes and HIV testing behaviors (38). The Behavioral Risk Factor Surveillance System has monitored a spectrum of health-related behaviors, including the use of an optional (for participating states) questionnaire on sexual behaviors (39). The Youth Risk Behavior Surveillance System (YRBSS) is a broad-spectrum health survey among teen-aged youth and has been used to monitor sexual behaviors, including condom use (40). The National Household Survey of Drug Abuse is a household survey of illicit drug use (41).

Each of these surveys, however, is targeted toward the "general population," usually meaning noninstitutionalized civilian persons who are accessible via a sampling frame that is defined by residence in a household, telephone ownership, or, for the YRBSS, school attendance. While these surveys are useful in broadly defining the prevalence of certain risk behaviors or in monitoring trends among the population at large, they may not be sufficiently inclusive or representative of those at highest risk for HIV infection to accurately track the behaviors among all groups of concern to public health specialists. For example, the limitation of general population-based sampling methods was brought to light in 1989 when the National Center for Health Statistics conducted a pilot test for a national household survey of HIV risk behaviors and HIV prevalence. In that instance, non-response rates among those presumably at highest risk for HIV substantially diminished the usefulness of this method (42).

The challenges in monitoring behaviors among "high-risk" populations include defining risk, identifying and accessing representative population groups that can be surveyed, defining a sampling frame, and obtaining sufficient response rates, particularly in settings where the population of interest may be apprehensive about providing sensitive information and distrustful of public health agencies. A variety of approaches have been used to address these challenges.

An important innovation in behavioral surveillance technique developed in response to HIV/AIDS draws on the tools of anthropology. The Young Men's Survey used anthropologic techniques to identify venues where young men who have sex with men (MSM) congregate, followed by the use of more formal sampling techniques, and combined with these active community-based outreach methods to identify and enroll participants from a variety of "nontraditional" survey sites, such as bars, parks, and other locations (43). Theoretically, this method could be modified and employed as an ongoing surveillance method.

In four major cities (Chicago, San Francisco, Los Angeles, and New York City) telephone surveys of health-related behaviors among MSM have been conducted by targeting neighborhoods where census and other data have identified those areas in which a high proportion of residents are MSM (44). Others have surveyed injection drug users at sites where needle exchange services are provided (45). State HIV prevention community-planning groups (see Chapter 3) have employed a variety of convenience-based, informal survey methods in their efforts to develop community profiles to assist local HIV prevention planning. This broad array of methods stretches the limits of the term "surveillance" but each has provided information that has been useful in either local or national decision making for HIV prevention programs.

Another approach to behavioral surveillance among at-risk populations is the use of proxy indicators of risk behaviors, such as trends in syphilis and gonorrhea rates. For example, declines in gonorrhea among men during the 1980s were broadly indicative of reductions in sexual risk behaviors among MSM following the recognition of the HIV/AIDS epidemic (46), while increases in gonorrhea among MSM during the late 1990s have been interpreted as an indicator of increases in sexual risk behaviors, attributed in part to "prevention fatigue" and lessened concerns about HIV in the era of highly active antiretroviral therapies (47,48,49). Similar increases in syphilis among MSM in some urban centers in the late 1990s and early 2000s, despite overall national declines in syphilis, further heighten concerns about increases in sexual risk behaviors (50,51). Another "proxy" measure of risk behaviors is provided by the Drug Abuse Warning Network (DAWN) (52). This surveillance system, sponsored by the Substance Abuse and Mental Health Services Administration, monitors trends in drug overdoses diagnosed at a national sample of U.S. emergency rooms. Trends in overdoses can reflect variations in the prevalence and modes (e.g., injection, snorting) of drug use, as well as changes in the price and purity of illicit drugs.

For diseases like HIV that are not uniformly distributed throughout the population but are relatively concentrated in at-risk population groups, general population surveys are useful but limited in their ability to track trends in behaviors that can lead to infection or disease. Because public health programs are heavily targeted toward high-risk groups, it is important that behavioral surveillance data be similarly geared to providing information that describes trends in risk behaviors within these groups. No single surveillance method is likely to be ideal, and, as characterized above, an approach that attempts to fill in as many pieces of the "mosaic" as possible is needed. In addition, new approaches may be required to survey high-risk groups, including community outreach that engenders the trust and participation of target populations. Innovations in behavioral surveillance techniques and approaches developed in response to HIV/AIDS will be useful in other public health circumstances, especially in situations involving marginalized populations or when health problems are disproportionately concentrated among high-risk groups.

Lesson 3: Active Collaboration among Public Health Stakeholders

Surveillance, particularly for conditions of high public health importance and visibility like HIV/AIDS, operates in the broad public health arena. As such, the public expects HIV/AIDS data to be as comprehensive and as accurate as possible (if not more comprehensive or accurate than possible), and public health agencies are held accountable for the answers that surveillance systems can or cannot provide. Although many public health agencies now routinely involve a mix of constituents in developing surveillance policies for HIV/AIDS, including program managers and advocates for those at greatest risk for HIV, the value of this approach was not fully appreciated earlier in the epidemic. In addition, public attitudes toward data collection, the methods of data collection, and the value of health statistics (e.g., perceptions of surveillance as "counting" versus "caring") can affect the options available to epidemiologists in conducting surveillance. Thus, it is essential for decisions about surveillance to be made with an understanding of the broader social context in which surveillance is conducted, allowing for the most effective approach to solving problems that require both epidemiologic and political[a] expertise. For this to be done effectively, skills and perspectives other than epidemiology need to be engaged, including expertise in public health program management, policy analysis, communications, community relations and certainly the perspective of those to be served by the intended public health effort. Two situations where this lesson was learned somewhat painfully for epidemiologists in the United States were the 1993 revision of the AIDS surveillance definition (53) and the events leading to CDC's discontinuation of the Survey of Childbearing Women.

The AIDS surveillance definition was developed shortly after the recognition of the syndrome in 1981 (54) and was revised in 1985 (55) and 1987 (56) in response to the discovery of HIV, the development of a serologic test for HIV infection, changing clinical practice, and increasing knowledge about the spectrum of HIV-related disease. Although relatively complicated, the definition had two

---

[a] The term *political* is not used here to refer to partisan politics but, rather, to the larger area of public interests and the processes used to resolve differences of opinion and perspective.

basic components: evidence of HIV infection (or absence of evidence of other known causes of immune dysfunction), combined with evidence of one or more "indicator" diseases associated with impaired immunity. With each of these revisions, CDC sought advice by convening consultations that were relatively small and primarily involved experts in HIV clinical care and epidemiology.

By the time the AIDS surveillance was revised again in 1993, CDC had convened multiple consultations of increasing size and visibility over a two-year period, including a public forum in September 1992 that was covered by national media outlets and featured speakers who represented traditional public health perspectives (e.g., health departments, clinical experts, professional organizations), as well as persons with HIV and representatives of various HIV advocacy organizations. Interest in the definition extended well beyond epidemiologists; it was the featured topic at an emotionally charged plenary session at the 1992 international conference on AIDS in Amsterdam; CDC offices had been picketed and occupied by demonstrators protesting the agency's then-current surveillance definition; hundreds of postcards had been mailed to CDC featuring a photograph of the agency's lead HIV epidemiologist with an image of a "bull's-eye" target superimposed on his forehead; and CDC's proposed revision had been subjected to an extended period of formal public review. Clearly, this was the first time in the history of U.S. public health where the criteria used for reporting of a notifiable disease had attracted such widespread interest. What happened between 1987 and 1993, and what was learned from this experience?

Four forces converged to shape the controversies and debates that surrounded the 1993 revision. The first force was economic. The AIDS surveillance definition had been adopted by the Social Security Administration in 1988 as a criterion for eligibility for certain benefits (7,8). Thus, whether an individual met the published surveillance criteria for AIDS directly affected the level of services that were available.

The second force was epidemiologic; by the late 1980s, racial and ethnic disparities in AIDS incidence had become more apparent, and noticeable shifts were occurring in the characteristics of persons reported with AIDS. During the 1980s an increasing percentage of cases were reported among persons exposed to HIV through injection drug use or through heterosexual contact, and an increasing proportion of cases were reported among women (57,58). Up to this time, the AIDS surveillance definition had focused on a set of illnesses that were typically seen only in persons with impaired immunity. These diseases were known as "opportunistic infections" because they caused disease only when presented with the "opportunity" occasioned by impaired immunity. However, as groups at prior increased risk for "nonopportunistic" infections (e.g., injection drug users) began to account for an increasing proportion of the HIV-infected population and as knowledge about the spectrum of HIV-related disease continued to improve, it became increasingly apparent that a broader array of more common infections could also occur with greater frequency or severity among persons with HIV. For example, injection drug users (IDUs) are at increased risk for bacterial sepsis and pneumonia, infections that are not hallmarks of immune dysfunction, and by the mid- to late 1980s, increased morbidity and mortality attributed to these nonopportunistic infections were observed among IDUs in parallel with the HIV epidemic (18,19). In addition, tuberculosis, a disease much more prevalent among members of racial and ethnic minority groups than among whites in the United States, was observed to be more frequent and severe among persons with HIV (59). Among women, candida vaginitis, a common gynecologic disorder, was found to be an early sign of HIV-related immune dysfunction (60), and data emerged that the risk of cervical cancer was heightened among women with HIV infection (61).

Thus, before 1993, it was possible for an HIV-infected person to have certain types of severe or even fatal HIV-related disease and not meet the AIDS surveillance criteria (62). As a result of epidemiologic shifts, there was an increasing number of people, disproportionately of minority race or ethnicity, with severe and often fatal HIV-related disease who were not eligible for certain health service benefits and who were not represented in AIDS surveillance, the nation's primary indicator for tracking the HIV epidemic. Furthermore, because the AIDS definition was not developed to be a primary measure of health service needs, many other individuals who were ill in the pre-AIDS spectrum of HIV disease were not yet eligible for services.

The third force was social. AIDS activism had emerged as a powerful force, primarily on behalf of improving treatment and services for people with HIV (63). In the activists' view, the AIDS surveillance definition was a barrier to services and one that disproportionately affected persons of minority race/ethnicity and women.

The fourth force was the continuing advance in HIV care. By the late 1980s, the relationship between progressive immune dysfunction and HIV-related disease was increasingly understood (64), and monitoring of the CD4+ T-lymphocyte count as a means of tracking immune status was becoming routine practice. This provided an opportunity to include in the surveillance definition a single laboratory-based measure of HIV immune dysfunction that was independent of specific indicator diseases (65).

Clearly, the forces that affected the proposed revision of the AIDS definition were shaped by concerns much more diverse and complicated than considerations of surveillance methods alone. However, epidemiologists who recognized that the surveillance definition needed another update were troubled by "nonsurveillance" or "secondary" uses (e.g., the adoption of the surveillance definition as a criterion for service eligibility) driving the surveillance discussion. Many argued that improved epidemiologic monitoring should guide the revision of the surveillance definition and that service agencies should develop separate criteria to determine eligibility for programs. Judgments about whether this position was wise or naive are likely to depend on one's perspective.

Epidemiologists were also troubled by the difficulty in achieving the right balance between sensitivity (ensuring that all persons with severe HIV-related disease were included in AIDS reports) and specificity (ensuring that persons reported with AIDS indeed had illness related to, and not merely coincident with, HIV infection) in expanding surveillance criteria, while avoiding making the definition much more complicated. CDC's initial proposal to expand the definition by including a measure of severe immune suppression (a CD4+ T-lymphocyte count < 200 cells/μl) (65) was not fully accepted, however, (a) because of concerns that not all HIV-infected persons would have access to CD4+ T-cell lymphocyte testing, (b) because of concerns that certain severe diseases could occur before this level of immune suppression, and (c) because it lacked both the symbolic and educational value of including additional diseases that were particularly common or severe in populations emerging as increasingly important in the epidemic, including injection drug users and women.

The final resolution of the debate included the addition of this immune-based measure, as well as three additional indicator diseases: recurrent bacterial pneumonia (a disease particularly common among HIV-infected drug injectors), pulmonary tuberculosis (a disease that interacted with HIV and disproportionately affected racial and ethnic minority populations), and cervical cancer (a condition linked to HIV infection among women) (53,66). This resolution took several years to achieve and could likely have been achieved sooner (and with much less angst) had surveillance experts more effectively engaged both advocates and representatives of agencies that employed the definition for "nonsurveillance" purposes earlier in the discussion. Further, had experts in other disciplines such as policy analysis and communications been more effectively involved in assessing surveillance policy, it is likely that they would have been able to affect a rapprochement across the activist and traditionalist perspectives sooner.

Another instructive episode in the "learning curve" of HIV/AIDS surveillance concerns the Survey of Childbearing Women (SCBW). The SCBW was the "crown jewel" among the unlinked seroprevalence surveys because it was the only survey that was population-based, meaning that its "denominator" (women delivering live-born infants) was a well-defined population group whose epidemiologic characteristics could be readily compared to the population at large, and it was conducted in nearly all states. By using newborns' blood left over from routine metabolic screening, it was possible to monitor the prevalence of passively acquired maternal HIV antibodies and, thus, the prevalence of HIV infection among U.S. women giving birth. In fact, the SCBW had been useful in heralding the increase in HIV among women and in highlighting the strikingly disproportionate burden of HIV among women of minority race or ethnicity (67). In addition, because the demographic characteristics of women giving birth could be described from birth certificates and because the representatitveness of HIV prevalence among childbearing women could be compared to all other women, it was possible for the SCBW to be used as an anchor in mathematical estimates of national HIV prevalence (68).

Since the outset of unlinked HIV surveys, the ethics of this survey method had been discussed and debated (29,69,70,71), but the preponderance of ethical thinking favored the use of this technique, as long as several conditions were met. Surveys should be conducted in settings where blood was routinely collected for other health purposes, where left-over specimens were available (i.e., no extra blood was collected for the purpose of the survey and there was no direct interaction with persons whose blood was tested), and all identifying information was removed from the specimens before HIV testing was done. In the parlance of federal human subjects research guidelines, unlinked HIV serosurveys were deemed not to involve "human subjects," a position that was affirmed by the Office of Protection against Research Risks of the U.S. Department of Health and Human Services in 1995 (72). This justification of unlinked HIV surveillance, however, was not more broadly shared when subsequent events led to heightened public attention to maternal and newborn HIV testing (32).

As with the AIDS surveillance definition, several forces combined to shape the fate of the SCBW—forces that epidemiologists alone were ill equipped to address and that public health agencies were not prepared to address effectively (32). In 1994, the National Institutes of Health announced the results of the Pediatric AIDS Clinical Trials Group Study 076, which documented that a regimen of zidovudine (AZT) given to HIV-infected pregnant women during the latter stages of pregnancy and during labor, combined with administration of a six-week course to their newborns, reduced the risk of maternal-to-infant HIV transmission by about two-thirds (73,74). The results of this study were followed by the issuance of guidelines from the U.S. Public Health Service that all pregnant women be routinely offered voluntary HIV counseling and testing and that all pregnant women found to be HIV-infected be offered the zidovudine regimen for themselves and their newborn infants (75,76). This was a departure from prior recommendations that emphasized risk assessment and offering of voluntary HIV counseling and testing only to those women deemed to be a high risk—a strategy that had proved ineffective because many women were unaware of their risk or because prenatal care providers were reluctant to discuss HIV.

In addition, there was a growing reaction against "AIDS exceptionalism," a term coined to describe and challenge prevailing attitudes that the public health response to HIV should substantially differ from the response to other sexually transmitted or communicable diseases (77). Manifested by calls for expanded mandatory HIV testing, particularly among pregnant women, persons who challenged exceptionalism argued that HIV testing during pregnancy and/or after birth should be more routine, like prenatal testing for syphilis or postnatal newborn screening for comparatively rare genetic and metabolic conditions (32).

Antiexceptionalism arguments were strengthened by epidemiologic evidence documenting that many cases of HIV infection among infants were first detected by the appearance of potentially fatal opportunistic illnesses such as *Pneumocystis carinii* pneumonia (PCP), an infection that is readily preventable through the use of prophylactic medications if an infant's exposure to maternal HIV infection is recognized, and that cases of HIV-associated PCP in infants had not declined as hoped (78). They were also strengthened by the increasing recognition that breast feeding presented a sizeable risk of postnatal maternal-to-infant transmission if the mother's infection was not recognized and artificial formulas were not used for infant feeding (79). Ultimately, though, the recognition that the risk of perinatal transmission could be substantially reduced if the mother's infection were diagnosed and the prophylactic zidovudine regimen used led to heightened calls for expanded HIV testing (32). On the other side of the argument, concerns from advocates that mandating HIV testing would "drive" many women from seeking prenatal care were lent force by the voices of infected women. These concerns were exacerbated by fears that those calling for expanded testing would take punitive action against women who declined testing or declined the use of the zidovudine regimen and by concerns that the ongoing pre- and postnatal health-care needs of HIV-infected women themselves would be overlooked as attention was focused on preventing infections in infants (32). Finally and perhaps most forcefully was the simple power of the argument, however misconstrued from the epidemiologists' perspective, that the "government" was testing babies for HIV and sending them home from the nursery without telling anyone, an argument that drew inevitable comparisons to the U.S. Public Health Service's infamous experiment on untreated syphilis among black men in Tuskegee, Alabama (32).

One of the great ironies in this debate is that it focused largely on the SCBW and on calls to "unblind" the survey. This was ironic because the benefits of learning about HIV infection for the mother and infant were much greater during pregnancy, allowing for the optimal use of therapy to prevent transmission, than after delivery. In addition, the survey had not been designed to serve as a clinical preventive screening program. Procedures for processing, batching, and testing specimens were not configured on a time frame that was clinically useful; in some states, the survey was based on testing a sample rather than all specimens. Further, the actual test that was used had been validated for surveillance purposes but not licensed for clinical use. In short, calls to "unblind" the survey amounted to a call for instituting a system of mandatory newborn testing. This put CDC in a difficult position because the ethical review and approval by its Institutional Review Board for the SCBW was conditional on the survey being anonymous. Also, state, not federal, government maintains the authority to mandate the use of newborn screening tests.

In the midst of the controversy, the federal government convened a multidis-ciplinary consultation involving individuals with positions on multiple sides of the debate, and, while the meeting participants endorsed continuation of the SCBW, the broader impact of the meeting was inconclusive; mounting opposi-tion to the SCBW in prominent media outlets and among political leaders, in-cluding members of Congress, resulted in the suspension of the survey in 1995. Opponents of the survey were dismayed by the absence of mandatory newborn testing for HIV; supporters of the survey were frustrated by the loss of a key measure of the impact of HIV among women (32). Congress subsequently man-dated that states document progress in achieving high levels of maternal HIV testing and set specific goals, which, if not met, would lead to requirements for mandatory newborn testing as a precondition for receiving Ryan White Care Act funds. CDC continues to recommend routine voluntary counseling and testing during pregnancy or during labor for those women who have not received pre-natal care. Acceptance of these recommendations has greatly increased over time, and rates of perinatal HIV transmission have fallen dramatically in the United States, although a small number of cases continue to occur, mainly in women who have not received prenatal care (80,81).

Looking back on this episode, it is arguable whether continuing the SCBW was a viable option, but it is possible that the situation could have been managed in a way that minimized frustration and lessened the considerable criticism lev-eled at the federal government and the public health community. With the 1993 revision of the AIDS surveillance, case definition, a workable and reasonable res-olution was achieved that ultimately enhanced both the credibility and the use-fulness of AIDS surveillance; the outcome with the SCBW was far less con-structive in terms of maintaining the ability of states and the federal government to track the HIV epidemic.

In both of these situations, however, there are common lessons. The key lesson is that epidemiologic and methodologic expertise is essential but not always suffi-cient for ensuring that public health surveillance is successfully managed. Multi-ple skills are needed and must be effectively marshaled to ensure that surveillance systems are meeting the needs of the full array of constituents and that systems have the ongoing support that is essential for both their relevance and their con-tinued ability to function. This requires outreach to all constituents, environmental scanning and anticipation of emerging public concerns as manifest in the media, political discourse, feedback from managers of prevention and care programs, and assessments from policy analysts and communications specialists. Public health managers and administrators charged with developing new surveillance systems should take these lessons to heart, remembering not only to maintain a sound sci-entific approach to public health surveillance but also to implement management structures that allow for an effective synthesis and use of insights from multiple disciplines, including—but obviously not limited to—epidemiology.

Lesson 4: Confidentiality of Health Information

Concerns about the confidentiality of surveillance information have been prominent in shaping the development of HIV and AIDS surveillance methods, procedures, and policies. Substantial ongoing effort has been invested by federal, state,
and local health departments to ensure the security and confidentiality of surveillance data, protecting against unauthorized access to and inappropriate use
of HIV/AIDS information. Given the sensitivity of the information included in
HIV/AIDS reports, protecting this information is essential to maintaining the trust
of affected communities and health-care providers and thus support for surveillance. Procedures established for protecting the confidentiality of HIV/AIDS surveillance data have served as a model for other surveillance systems.

This strong record of confidentiality protection has not always been viewed as
constructive. The strict boundaries around HIV surveillance data have been
viewed at times, even within health departments, as a barrier to good public health
practice. For example, in some states, strict procedures for protecting the confidentiality of HIV/AIDS case reports have hindered collaboration between HIV
and tuberculosis program staff in providing comprehensive preventive services
to clients, even though the two infections often intersect in the same populations
and individuals. From the perspective of those responsible for managing information systems, the disease-specific "stovepipe" data management systems ex-
emplified by HIV/AIDS surveillance have been viewed as a hindrance to more
comprehensive, client- rather than disease-based information management across
public health programs. Nonetheless, the HIV/AIDS experience has served to
highlight the critical importance of confidentiality as states seek to develop more
integrated public health data systems.

Despite the strong record of health departments in protecting AIDS surveillance data, concerns about potential breaks in the protection of confidentiality
have been a major obstacle to states' efforts in adopting name-based HIV reporting over the past fifteen years (82,83). Discussions with those concerned
about confidentially of HIV/AIDS surveillance data demonstrate two key themes
regarding the public perception of the confidentiality of medical and public health
records in general. The first theme is that many in the public do not distinguish
between different branches of government or different agencies within government, if or when confidentiality is threatened. Thus, if a legislator makes a dis-
paraging remark about a group of individuals at risk for HIV infection, that can
lead to heightened concerns, particularly among members of that group, about
the ability of an agency in another government branch (e.g., the executive) to
protect confidentiality. This can manifest in statements such as, "We know you
in public health are committed to protecting confidentiality, but how can we be
assured that someone in another branch of government won't seek to override
you?" The second theme is that violations of confidentiality in one sector (e.g.,

a failure to protect confidentiality at a private hospital) can affect community attitudes about confidentiality in a completely different sector (e.g., a public health department responsible for surveillance) holding sensitive health information. Such perceptions can have a powerful influence on the public and on the legislative governance that shapes surveillance practice. As such, these concerns can only be offset by sustained and effective advocacy for, and management of, security and confidentiality procedures by public health agencies.

While the experience with HIV/AIDS surveillance has served to highlight issues surrounding confidentiality, the importance of public concerns about privacy and confidentiality clearly reflect deeply held values about personal health information, well beyond HIV/AIDS surveillance. This was evident at the time that regionalized data systems were proposed as part of health-care reforms during the early years of the Clinton administration (84) and during the development of health data privacy guidelines by the Department of Health and Human Services as mandated by the Health Insurance Portability and Accountability Act (HIPAA) of 1996 (85,86). As surveillance systems become increasingly automated and as public discussions, such as the one that accompanied the development of the HIPAA-mandated rules, draw increasing attention to personal data collection by government agencies, it is likely that public concerns about privacy of health data will continue to shape public policies that define how surveillance is conducted.

Conclusions

Each of these "lessons learned" through the HIV/AIDS surveillance experience—the importance of using multiple surveillance methods for monitoring complex diseases; the need for focused behavioral surveillance when health problems have a behavioral dimension and disproportionately affect high-risk population groups; the importance of a multidisciplinary approach that includes both epidemiology and other public health perspectives when surveillance intersects with broader public concerns; and the critical importance of respecting privacy and protecting confidentiality while meeting public health responsibilities—are lessons that are not unique to the prevention and control of HIV/AIDS. Yet, undeniably, the HIV/AIDS epidemic has focused attention on the importance of these lessons in a unique way, drawing surveillance from the background of public health practice and propelling it into the forefront. The impact of HIV/AIDS on groups such as men who have sex with men and injection drug users, who have long been stigmatized by society, its disproportionate impact on persons of minority race or ethnicity, the active and sometimes boisterous involvement of advocacy groups, and the striking advances in HIV prevention and treatment—all have combined to place unprecedented and urgent demands on the planners and managers of surveillance systems.

These lessons will become increasingly relevant for broader public health practice as public health agencies address health conditions that are characterized by a spectrum that extends from pre-disease risk behaviors or exposures to asymptomatic and later life-threatening disease, regardless of whether the diseases are of infectious or noninfectious etiology. For example, diabetes is a complex disease with a long-term course and multiple complications, and CDC's comprehensive approach to diabetes surveillance is based on synthesis of data from many sources (87). These lessons will also be relevant as the diseases addressed by public health agencies arouse broad public interest and, by extension, media and political interest. The cluster of anthrax cases related to bioterrorism in 2001 (88) provides a recent illustration of the complexities of managing a public health activity, including accompanying surveillance systems, under intense public scrutiny. The tremendous interest in anthrax surveillance data and the attention of a frightened nation to their interpretation and communication, along with other scientific information, highlights the importance of integrating epidemiologic expertise with other disciplines, particularly public health communications (89). There was a time when epidemiology was considered as *the* basic science of public health, but that view has been replaced by a vision of public health that emphasizes the importance of collaboration across disciplines (90). Experience with HIV/AIDS demonstrates that epidemiology is just one of many disciplines essential to effectively managing public health surveillance.

References

1. Buehler JW: Surveillance. In Rothman KJ and Greenland S (eds.): *Modern Epidemiology*, 2nd ed. Lippincott-Raven, Philadelphia, 1998, pp. 435–457.
2. Centers for Disease Control and Prevention: Updated guidelines for evaluating public health surveillance systems: recommendations from the guidelines working group. *Morb Mortal Wkly Rep* 50(RR13): 13–24, 2001.
3. Centers for Disease Control and Prevention: *Pneumocystis* pneumonia—Los Angeles. *Morb Mortal Wkly Rep* 30: 250–252, 1981.
4. Fleming PL, Wortley PM, Karon JM, Decock KM, and Janssen RS. Tracking the HIV epidemic: current issues, future challenges. *Am J Public Health* 90: 1037–1041, 2000.
5. Centers for Disease Control and Prevention: *HIV/AIDS Surveillance Report* 13(1): 36–40, 2001. URL: http://www.cdc.gov/hiv/stats/.
6. Institute of Medicine, Committee on HIV Prevention Strategies in the United States: *No Time to Lose, Getting More from HIV Prevention.* National Academy Press, Washington, DC, 2001, pp. 28–32.
7. HIV/AIDS Bureau, Health Resources and Service Administration, U.S. Department of Health and Human Services: Ryan White Care Act, History. URL: http://hrsa.gov/history.htm.
8. Social Security Administration: Supplemental security income for the aged, blind and disabled; presumptive disability and presumptive blindness; categories of impairments—AIDS. *Federal Register* 53: 3739–3742, 1988.

 9. U.S. Congress, Office of Technology Assessment. *The CDC's Case Definition for AIDS: Implications of the Proposed Revision—Background Paper*, (OTA-BP-H-89). Government Printing Office, Washington DC, 1992.

10. Fordyce EJ, Sambula S, and Stoneburner R. Mandatory reporting of human immunodeficiency virus testing would deter blacks and Hispanics from being tested (letter). *JAMA* 262: 349, 1989.

11. Hecht FM, Chesney M, Lehman JS, et al.: Does HIV reporting by name deter testing? *AIDS* 14: 1801–1808, 2000.

12. Janssen RS, Satten GA, Stramer SL, et al.: New testing strategy to detect early HIV-1 infection for use in incidence estimates and for clinical prevention purposes. *JAMA* 280: 42–48, 1998 (see erratum: *JAMA* 281: 1893, 1999).

13. Rosenberg PS: Scope of the AIDS epidemic in the United States. *Science* 270: 1372–1375, 1995.

14. Karon JM, Khare M, and Rosenberg PS: The current status of methods for estimating the prevalence of human immunodeficiency virus infection in the United States of America. *Stat Med* 17: 127–142, 1998.

15. Sumartojo E: Structural factors in HIV/AIDS prevention: concepts, examples, and implications for research. *AIDS* 14(Suppl 1): S3–10, 2000.

16. Valdiserri RO: HIV/AIDS stigma: an impediment to public health [editorial]. *Am J Public Health* 92: 5–6, 2002.

17. Chamberland ME, Allen JR, Monroe JM, et al.: Acquired immunodeficiency syndrome in New York City: evaluation of an active surveillance system. *JAMA* 254: 383–387, 1985.

18. Stoneburner RL, Des Jarlais DC, Benezra D, et al.: A larger spectrum of severe HIV-1-related disease in intravenous drug users in New York City. *Science* 242: 916–919, 1988.

19. Centers for Disease Control and Prevention: Increase in pneumonia mortality among young adults and the HIV epidemic—New York City, United States. *Morb Mortal Wkly Rep* 37: 593–596, 1988.

20. Buehler JW, Berkelman RL, and Stehr-Green JK: The completeness of AIDS surveillance. *J Acquir Immune Defic Syndr* 5: 257–264, 1992.

21. Rosenberg L, Buehler JW, Morgan MW, et al.: The completeness of AIDS case reporting, 1988: a multisite collaborative surveillance project. *Am J Public Health* 82: 1495–1499, 1992.

22. Caldwell MB, Mascola L, Smith W, et al.: Biologic, foster, and adoptive parents: care givers of children perinatally exposed to human immunodeficiency virus in the United States. *Pediatrics* 90: 603–607, 1992.

23. Farizo KM, Buehler JW, Chamberland M, et al.: Spectrum of disease in persons with human immunodeficiency virus infection in the United States. *JAMA* 267: 1798–1805, 1992.

24. Buehler JW, Diaz T, Hersch BS, and Chu SY: The Supplement to HIV-AIDS Surveillance Project: an approach for monitoring HIV risk behaviors. *Public Health Rep* 111(Suppl. 1): 133–137, 1996.

25. Centers for Disease Control and Prevention: HIV testing among populations at risk for HIV infection—nine states, November 1995–December 1996. *Morb Mortal Wkly Rep* 47: 1086–1091, 1998; (see also Erratum *Morb Mortal Wkly Rep* 49: 762–763, 2000).

26. Safran M and Wilson R: Surveillance of HIV knowledge, attitudes, beliefs, and behaviors in the general population. *Public Health Rep* 111(Suppl. 1): 123–128, 1996.

27. Anderson J: CDC data systems collecting behavioral data on HIV counseling and testing. *Public Health Rep* 111(Suppl. 1): 129–132, 1996.
28. Centers for Disease Control and Prevention: CDC guidelines for national human immunodeficiency virus case surveillance, including monitoring for human immunodeficiency virus infection and acquired immunodeficiency virus infection and acquired immunodeficiency syndrome. *Morb Mortal Wkly Rep* 48(RR13): 1–28, 1999.
29. Dondero TJ, Pappaioanou M, and Curran JW: Monitoring the levels and trends of HIV infection: the Public Health Service's HIV surveillance program. *Public Health Rep* 103: 213–220, 1988.
30. Centers for Disease Control and Prevention: *National HIV Prevalence Surveys: Summary of Results. Data from Serosurveillance activities through 1989* (HIV/CID/9-90/006). Centers for Disease Control, Public Health Service, Atlanta, 1990.
31. Centers for Disease Control and Prevention: *National HIV Prevalence Surveys: 1997 Summary.* Centers for Disease Control and Prevention, Atlanta, 1998, pp. 1–25, URL: http://www.cdc.gov/hiv/pubs/hivsero.htm.
32. Ogden LL: How politics undermines good science: public health policy on HIV/AIDS, politics, and the press. Master's thesis, John F. Kennedy School of Government, Harvard University, 1998.
33. Rutherford GW, Schwarcz SK, and McFarland W: Surveillance for incident HIV infection: new technology and new opportunities (review). *J Acquir Immune Defic Syndr* 25(Suppl): S115–S119, 2000.
34. Des Jarlais DC, Marmor M, Paone D, et al.: HIV incidence among injecting drug users in New York City syringe-exchange programmes. *Lancet* 348: 987–991, 1996.
35. Laird C: HIV infections on rise in SF. *Bay Area Reporter*, January 26, 2001. URL: http://www.aegis.com/news/bar/2001/BR010115.html.
36. Centers for Disease Control and Prevention: *Addressing Emerging Infectious Disease Threats: A Prevention Strategy for the United States.* U.S. Department of Health and Human Services, Public Health Service, CDC, Atlanta, 1994. URL: http://www.cdc.gov/ncidod/publications/eid_plan/downstra.htm.
37. Mosher WD and Pratt WF. *AIDS-Related Behavior among Women 15–44 Years of Age: United States, 1988 and 1990.* Advance data from vital and health statistics; no. 239. National Center for Health Statistics, Hyattsville, MD, 1993. URL: http://www.cdc.gov/nchs/data/ad/ad239.pdf.
38. Centers for Disease Control and Prevention: HIV counseling and testing services from public and private providers—United States, 1990. *Morb Mortal Wkly Rep* 41: 743,749–752, 1992.
39. Centers for Disease Control and Prevention: Prevalence of risk behaviors for HIV infection among adults—United States, 1997. *Morb Mortal Wkly Rep* 50: 262–265, 2001.
40. Centers for Disease Control and Prevention: Trends in HIV-related sexual risk behaviors among high school students—selected U.S. cities, 1991–1997. *Morb Mortal Wkly Rep* 48:440–443, 1999.
41. Substance Abuse and Mental Health Services Administration: Summary of Findings from the 2000 National Household Survey on Drug Abuse. URL: http://www.samhsa.gov/oas/NHSDA/2kNHSDA/2kNHSDA.htm.
42. Centers for Disease Control and Prevention: Current trends pilot study of a household survey to determine HIV seroprevalence. *Morb Mortal Wkly Rep* 40: 1–5, 1991.
43. Valleroy LA, MacKellar DA, Karon JM, et al.: HIV prevalence and associated risks in young men who have sex with men. *JAMA* 284: 198–204, 2000.

44. Stall R, Pollack L, Mills T, et al.: Use of antiretroviral therapies among HIV-infected men who have sex with men: a household-based sample of four major American cities. *Am J Public Health* 91(5): 767–773, 2001.

45. Des Jarlais DC, Paone, D, Milliken J, et al.: Audio-computer interviewing to measure risk behaviour for HIV among injecting drug users: a quasi-randomised trial. *Lancet* 353: 1657–1661, 1999.

46. Centers for Disease Control and Prevention: Declining rates of rectal and pharyngeal gonorrhea among males—New York City. *Morb Mortal Wkly Rep* 33: 295–297, 1984.

47. Centers for Disease Control and Prevention: Resurgent bacterial sexually transmitted disease among men who have sex with men—King County, Washington, 1997–1999. *Morb Mortal Wkly Rep* 48: 773–777, 1999.

48. Centers for Disease Control and Prevention: Increases in unsafe sex and rectal gonorrhea among men who have sex with men—San Francisco, California, 1994–1997. *Morb Mortal Wkly Rep* 48: 45–48, 1999.

49. Fox KK, del Rio C, Holmes KK, et al.: Gonorrhea in the HIV era: a reversal in trends among men who have sex with men. *Am J Public Health* 91: 959–964, 2001.

50. Centers for Disease Control and Prevention: *Sexually Transmitted Disease Surveillance, 2000.* U.S. Department of Health and Human Services, Centers for Disease Control and Prevention, Atlanta, 2001.

51. Centers for Disease Control and Prevention: Outbreak of syphilis among men who have sex with men—Southern California, 2000. *Morb Mortal Wkly Rep* 50: 117–120, 2001.

52. Substance Abuse and Mental Health Services Administration: Drug Abuse Warning Network (DAWN). URL: http://www.samhsa.gov/oas/dawn.htm.

53. Centers for Disease Control and Prevention: Revised classification system for HIV infection and expanded surveillance case definition for AIDS among adolescents and adults. *Morb Mortal Wkly Rep* 41(RR17): 1–19, 1992.

54. Centers for Disease Control and Prevention: Current trends update on acquired immune deficiency syndrome (AIDS)—United States. *Morb Mortal Wkly Rep* 31: 507–508, 513–514, 1982.

55. Centers for Disease Control and Prevention: Current trends revision of the case definition of acquired immunodeficiency syndrome for national reporting—United States. *Morb Mortal Wkly Rep* 34: 373–375, 1985.

56. Centers for Disease Control and Prevention: Revision of the CDC surveillance case definition for acquired immunodeficiency syndrome. *Morb Mortal Wkly Rep* 36(Suppl. 1S), pp. 1S–15S, 1987.

57. Centers for Disease Control and Prevention: Current trends first 100,000 cases of acquired immunodeficiency syndrome—United States. *Morb Mortal Wkly Rep* 38: 561–563, 1989.

58. Centers for Disease Control and Prevention: Current trends AIDS in women—United States. *Morb Mortal Wkly Rep* 39: 845–846, 1990.

59. Chaisson RE and Slutkin G: Tuberculosis and human immunodeficiency virus infection [review]. *J Infectious Dis* 159: 96–100, 1989.

60. Rhoads JL, Wright DC, Redfield RR, and Burke DS: Chronic vaginal candidiasis in women with human immunodeficiency virus infection. *JAMA* 257: 3105–3107, 1987.

61. Henry MJ, Stanley MW, Cruikshank S, and Carson L: Association of human immunodeficiency virus-induced immunosuppression with human papillomavirus infection and cervical intraepithelial neoplasia. *Am J Obstet Gynecol* 160: 352–353, 1989.

62. Farizo KF, Buehler JW, Chamberland ME, et al.: Spectrum of disease in persons with

human immunodeficiency virus infection in the United States. *JAMA* 267: 1798–1805, 1992.

63. Valdiserri RO: HIV/AIDS's contribution to community mobilization. In Valdiserri RO (ed.): *Dawning Answers: How the HIV/AIDS Epidemic Has Helped to Strengthen Public Health.* Oxford University Press, New York, pp. 56–75.

64. Phillips A, Lee CA, Elford J, et al.: Prediction of progression to AIDS by analysis of CD4 lymphocyte counts in a haemophilic cohort. *AIDS* 3: 737–741, 1989.

65. Buehler JW: The surveillance definition for AIDS [editorial]. *Am J Public Health* 82: 1462–1464, 1992.

66. Buehler JW and Ward JW. A new definition for AIDS surveillance. *Ann Intern Med* 118: 390–392, 1993.

67. Gwinn M, Pappaioanou M, George JR, et al.: Prevalence of HIV infection in child-bearing women in the United States: surveillance using newborn blood samples. *JAMA* 265: 1704–1708, 1991.

68. Centers for Disease Control and Prevention: Projections of the number of persons diagnosed with AIDS and the number of immunosuppressed HIV-infected persons—United States, 1992–1994. *Morb Mortal Wkly Rep* 41(RR-18): 1–29, 1992.

69. Isaacman SH: HIV surveillance testing: taking advantage of the disadvantaged. *Am J Public Health* 83: 597–598, 1993.

70. Buehler JW, Petersen LR, Ward JW, and Valdiserri RO: Defending HIV seroprevalence surveys (letter). *Am J Public Health* 84: 319–320, 1994.

71. Bayer R: The ethics of blinded HIV surveillance testing [letter]. *Am J Public Health* 83: 496–497, 1993.

72. Office of Protection from Research Risks, U.S. Department of Health and Human Services: Evaluation of Human Subjects Protections in Research Conducted by the Centers for Disease Control and Prevention and the Agency for Toxic Substances and Disease Registry. Report to CDC issued July 28, 1995.

73. National Institute of Allergy and Infectious Diseases: *Clinical Alert: Important Therapeutic Information on the Benefit of Zidovudine for the Prevention of the Transmission of HIV from Mother to Infant.* National Institutes of Health, National Institute of Allergy and Infectious Diseases, Bethesda, MD, 1994.

74. Connor EM, Sperling RS, Gelber R, et al.: Reduction of maternal–infant transmission of human immunodeficiency virus type 1 with zidovudine treatment. *N Engl J Med* 331: 1173–1180, 1994.

75. Centers for Disease Control and Prevention: Recommendations of the U.S. Public Health Service task force on the use of zidovudine to reduce perinatal transmission of human immunodeficiency virus. *Morb Mortal Wkly Rep* 43(RR11): 1–20, 1994.

76. Centers for Disease Control and Prevention: U.S. Public Health Service recommendations for human immunodeficiency virus counseling and voluntary testing for pregnant women. *Morb Mortal Wkly Rep* 44(RR7): 1–15, 1995.

77. Bayer R: Public health policy and the AIDS epidemic: an end to HIV exceptionalism? *N Engl J Med* 324: 1500–1504, 1991.

78. Simonds RJ, Lindegren ML, Thomas P, et al.: Prophylaxis against *Pneumocystis carinii* pneumonia among children with perinatally acquired human immunodeficiency virus infection in the United States. *N Engl J Med* 332: 786–790, 1995.

79. Dunn DT, Newell ML, Ades AE, and Peckham CS: Risk of human immunodeficiency virus type 1 transmission through breastfeeding. *Lancet* 340: 585–588, 1992.

80. Lindegren ML, Byers RH Jr, Thomas P, Davis SF, Caldwell B, Rogers M, Gwinn M, Ward JW, and Fleming PL: Trends in perinatal transmission of HIV/AIDS in the United States. *JAMA* 282: 531–538, 1999.

81. CDC. Successful implementation of perinatal HIV prevention guidelines, a multistate surveillance evaluation. *Morb Mortal Wkly Rep* 50(RR06): 17–28, 2001.
82. Gostin LO and Webber DW: HIV infection and AIDS in the public health and health care systems: the role of law and litigation. *JAMA* 279: 1108–1113, 1998.
83. Centers for Disease Control and Prevention: Evaluation of HIV case surveillance through the use of non-name unique identifiers—Maryland and Texas, 1994–1996. *Morb Mortal Wkly Rep* 46: 1254–1258, 1271, 1998
84. Donaldson M (ed): *Regional Health Databases, Health Services Research, and Confidentiality. Summary of an Invitational Workshop at the Institute of Medicine: National Implications of the Development of Regional Health Database Organizations, January 31–February 1, 1994.* Institute of Medicine, Washington, DC, 1994.
85. Office for Civil Rights: *National Standards to Protect the Privacy of Personal Health Information.* U.S. Department of Health and Human Services, Washington, DC, 2000. URL: http://www.hhs.gov/ocr/hipaa/
86. Gostin LO: National health information privacy: regulations under the Health Insurance Portability and Accountability Act. *JAMA* 285: 3015–3021, 2001.
87. Centers for Disease Control and Prevention, Diabetes Public Health Resource: Statistics, Diabetes Surveillance, 1999; Appendix, Data Sources and Limitations. URL: http://www.cdc.gov/diabetes/statistics/survl99/chap1/appendix.htm.
88. Centers for Disease Control and Prevention: Update: investigation of bioterrorism-related anthrax, 2001. *Morb Mortal Wkly Rep* 50: 1008–1010, 2001.
89. Stolberg SG and Miller J: Bioterror role an uneasy fit for disease centers. *New York Times*, November 11, 2001. URL: http://www.nytimes.com/2001/11/11/national/11CDC.html.
90. Savitz DA, Poole C, and Miller WC. Reassessing the role of epidemiology in public health. *Am J Public Health* 89: 1158–1161, 1999.

3

HIV/AIDS' Contribution to Community Mobilization and Health Planning Efforts

RONALD O. VALDISERRI

Public health can be described as an "organized community effort to address the public interest in health by applying scientific and technical knowledge to prevent disease and promote health" (1). The U.S. Constitution makes clear that government assumes the responsibility for protecting community health (2). At the federal level, the ability to tax, spend, and regulate interstate commerce is the most important power that government has at its disposal to prevent injury and disease and to promote the public's health (3). But it is state and local governments that have the predominant role in population-based health services, based on the "inherent authority of the state to enact laws and promulgate regulations to protect, preserve, and promote the health, safety . . . and general welfare of the people" (3).

Although government plays a central role in assuring public health, this mission is also shared by other public- and by private-sector organizations (1). The history of public health practice contains numerous examples of nongovernmental organizations (NGOs) acting to prevent disease and promote health in a variety of domains, including sanitary reform, maternal and child health, tuberculosis control, the prevention of sexually transmitted diseases, and the promotion of cardiovascular health (4,5,6,7). Predictably, NGOs play a major role in HIV prevention (8,9) and care (10), both in the United States and internationally (11).

Essential Public Health Services

In contrast to medical care, which focuses on individuals, public health addresses the health needs and conditions of populations (12). Promoting health and preventing disease at a population level encompasses a variety of activities that are supported by multiple disciplines and are carried out in diverse venues. The breadth of these activities can be described under the rubric of ten essential public health services (13), which range from monitoring community health status to evaluating the effectiveness of population-based health services (Table 3–1).

Public health advocates lament that they are often faced with "genuine misunderstanding of the nature and benefits of public health" (14), and surveys of the general public indicate substantial gaps in understanding and attitudes about public health (15). A 1996 survey of some 4,800 adults in California revealed that most respondents identified activities such as ensuring food and water safety as "top priorities" for public health, but fewer than one-third of them recognized the importance of essential public health functions such as collecting community health data and monitoring community health trends (16).

In part, society's fragmented perceptions of public health may reflect the realities of resource allocation; the vast majority of national U.S. health spending goes to support personal health-care. In 1999, approximately 87.4 percent of total U.S. health expenditures ($1,057.7 billion) was spent on personal health-care; 5.9 percent ($72 billion) was for "program administration and the net cost of private health insurance," and 3.3 percent ($39.8 billion) was for "research and construction." Only 3.4 percent ($41.1 billion) of the total 1999 U.S. national health expenditure was spent on "government public health activities" (17).

Even within the realm of public health spending, allocations vary substantially across activities and services. Nine states, developing detailed estimates of their

TABLE 3–1. Essential Public Health Services

Monitor health status to identify community health problems
Diagnose and investigate health problems and health hazards in the community
Inform, educate, and empower people about health issues
Mobilize community partnerships to identify and solve health problems
Develop policies and plans that support individual and community health efforts
Enforce laws and regulations that protect health and ensure safety
Link people to needed personal health services and assure the provision of health care when otherwise unavailable
Assure a competent public health and personal health care workforce
Evaluate effectiveness, accessibility, and quality of personal and population-based health services
Conduct research for new insights and innovative solutions to health problems

Source: P Lee and D Paxman, Reinventing public health, *Annu Rev Public Health* 18: 1–35, 1997.

1995 public health expenditures, estimated that 69 percent of their total public health spending was devoted to ensuring the provision of medical care when it was otherwise unavailable (a widely recognized responsibility of public health) and that only 31 percent went to population-based health services (18). The largest proportion of the population-based expenditures supported the enforcement of laws and regulations (26 percent), the diagnosis and investigation of health problems and health hazards in the community (17 percent), and informing, educating, and empowering people about health issues (16 percent) (18). Much smaller levels of expenditure were reported for the essential public health functions of mobilizing community partnerships to identify and solve health problems and of developing policies and plans to support individual and community health efforts (18).

While community mobilization, health planning, and priority setting may not spring to mind when the term "public health" is invoked, they are nevertheless essential to achieving sound public health outcomes. This chapter will review the ongoing influence of the HIV/AIDS epidemic on community mobilization and health planning efforts, including planning and priority setting related to public health research, and will enumerate lessons learned that apply to other fields of public health.

Community Mobilization and HIV/AIDS

Community mobilization in the face of HIV/AIDS is not a unique event in the annals of public health; many community responses to other infectious diseases and assorted health threats have occurred (19,20). Further, community mobilization is not specific to the field of public health. As described by Minkler and Wallerstein, community mobilization is closely related to the concept of community organization, a "process by which community groups are helped to identify common problems or goals, mobilize resources, and in other ways develop and implement strategies for reaching the goals they collectively have set" (21). Community organizing can have a number of explicit goals beyond health promotion, ranging from the political and the social to the economic (20,21).

What, then, are the unique dimensions of community mobilization in response to HIV/AIDS, and how have these circumstances and experiences influenced public health's capacity to mobilize community partnerships to identify and respond to other health problems? Freudenberg and Zimmerman observe that "the community response to AIDS prevention and services represented a qualitatively different level of involvement than previous reactions to other health conditions" (19). Similarly, Bastos notes that while AIDS wasn't "the first disease to generate the formation of patient groups," the degree of "patient-based activism that grew in the fight against AIDS was unprecedented" (22). How can these qualitative differences be explained?

Community mobilization around HIV/AIDS occurred first in the gay community. In the epidemic's early years, it was estimated that one out of every twenty-five gay men in New York's Greenwich Village "was living with or had already died of AIDS" (23). The prevalence of infection among San Francisco's gay community was even more staggering. By 1985, nearly three-quarters of a cohort of 6,875 homosexual and bisexual men, recruited in San Francisco between 1978 and 1980 to participate in a hepatitis B virus study, were found to be infected with the virus causing AIDS (24). To put this rate in perspective, consider that at the end of 1999, in Botswana, the country believed to have the highest known HIV seroprevalence rate in the world, it was estimated that nearly 36 percent of the adult population was infected with HIV (25).

The purpose of this comparison is not meant to minimize the burden of AIDS in Africa, which is horrific, or to elevate the suffering of one community over another. Instead, these data are presented to place the gay community's response to AIDS in context. The enormity of the AIDS threat experienced by various communities of gay men across the United States, coupled with the inadequacy of society's initial response to the epidemic (26,27), fueled a sense of urgency and purpose. As Andriote notes, "in terms of sheer volume of sickness and death—of mostly young people—the experience of gay Americans is unprecedented, particularly in an age when we thought medical science had conquered infectious disease" (23). Thus, an organizing premise of this discussion is that the magnitude of the AIDS threat experienced by gay communities in the first years of the epidemic led to an enhanced awareness of the problem by those communities, and to the accelerated development of community strategies to mobilize resources and to intervene—often in advance of organized public health efforts to do the same. Further, it is posited that early community mobilization efforts in response to AIDS have left a lasting mark on ongoing advocacy surrounding HIV disease and have influenced advocacy for other public health and medical concerns as well.

Advocacy to Reduce Death and Disability

Public health advocacy is a useful lens through which to explore HIV/AIDS' contribution to community mobilization approaches. Christoffel defines it as "advocacy that is intended to reduce death or disability" and conceptualizes three stages in its development: information, strategy, and action (28). The information stage includes activities that describe and quantify the scope of the public health problem. Coalitions to work on the problem often are mobilized during the strategy phase, and specific strategies are implemented during the action stage.

While community mobilization is not unique to HIV/AIDS, what is noteworthy is the magnitude of the community response and the central role of people living with HIV/AIDS (PLWHAs) in shaping public health practice and policy responses to the epidemic (29). Some analysts assert that AIDS activists "forced a major shift in the old public health approach to infectious disease control" (30), "helped democratize health policy" (30), and added a "jarring new dimension to what was previously a genteel dialogue between patient advocates and clinicians, researchers, and policy makers" (31).

Leaders from the communities of gay men suffering from this mysterious new disease were quick to take action. Early examples of community mobilization in response to AIDS in the United States include the formation of the Gay Mens Health Crisis (GMHC) in New York City and the Kaposi Sarcoma Education and Research Foundation in San Francisco (later renamed the San Francisco AIDS Foundation); both organizations were established in 1982 (32). These organizations and others like them engaged in fund raising, volunteer recruitment and training, and the provision of education and care services—including assigning "buddies" to clients who were too ill to take care of their own practical support needs (22).

As described in Chapter 1 of this volume, communities were typically at the forefront of early AIDS prevention efforts, often in advance of government responses. Brochure development, condom distribution, even the establishment of local information hotlines were all spearheaded by "storefront activists and concerned doctors" from affected communities (33). But as the epidemic progressed, advocacy efforts moved beyond the immediate service needs of client education, care, and support. Particularly critical was the need to engage individuals outside of the gay community in the fight against AIDS—to make them aware of the dangers posed by the virus and to mobilize their support for requisite prevention, research, and treatment.

An especially unique approach to mobilizing communities to respond to the threat of AIDS can be found in the NAMES Project AIDS Memorial Quilt. Rather than relying on dry statistics and bloodless epidemiologic reports to help people understand the devastating effects of AIDS, the quilt is composed of over 40,000 handmade panels that memorialize persons lost to AIDS. Panels are contributed by family members, friends, and colleagues. First started by Cleve Jones and a group of volunteers in San Francisco in 1987, the quilt has grown to become a globally recognized symbol of the epidemic and a powerful tool for creating awareness of it (34). As one observer wrote in 1991: "Although I was aware of AIDS and the statistics broadcast on the news, viewing the Quilt shocked me into dealing with those numbers on a more personal level. To think of each panel as a representation of other human beings . . . forced me to realize the true tragedy of this crisis" (34:291).

A very different approach to HIV/AIDS community mobilization came into prominence in 1987, when activist and playwright Larry Kramer formed the AIDS Coalition to Unleash Power (ACT UP) in New York City (35). ACT UP was formed in reaction to "the sluggish response of the medical establishment to the

AIDS crisis"; its first order of business was "to increase access to new drugs for people with AIDS" (35). In addition to its strong treatment agenda, ACT UP also maintained a prominent focus on prevention, especially efforts to encourage safer sex and "safer drug use" (i.e., providing unfettered access to sterile injection equipment for injecting drug users who chose not to stop injecting).

With a mission statement that defined the organization as "united in anger and committed to direct action to end the AIDS epidemic," ACT UP's tactics often involved public displays of civil disobedience (35). Predictably, many found ACT UP's confrontational approach off-putting. Nevertheless, analysts have credited ACT UP and other AIDS activists with influencing the Food and Drug Administration (FDA) to "streamline" its procedures for drug approval (30,36) and with pressuring manufacturers to lower the price of antiretroviral treatments (31). And certainly, ACT UP's highly publicized and often provocative tactics related to safer sex and "safer drug use" brought these prevention issues to the consciousness of Americans who might have been unaware of them or otherwise refused to confront them.

Another significant manifestation of community frustration with the slow government process of AIDS drug approval and release was the formation of "community-based" trials. Described as a development "unprecedented in the history of medicine" (37), these collaborations between persons with AIDS and their physicians aimed to create scientifically valid and ethically sound trials of "practical treatment options" that might not otherwise be tested, trials that were designed to get results more rapidly than traditional research approaches (37). By 1987, community-based groups in New York City (Community Research Initiative) and San Francisco (Community Consortium) had been established and had begun to conduct clinical trials on the effectiveness of aerosolized pentamidine as a prophylactic treatment for Pneumocystis carinii pneumonia (38). Based on results from the New York and San Francisco trials (38,39,40), the Food and Drug Administration approved a "treatment IND" (investigational new drug) for aerosol pentamidine as both primary and secondary prophylaxis for *Pneumocystis carinii* pneumonia (41).

The first Presidential Commission on HIV, recognizing the potential value of community-based clinical trials, directed the National Institute of Allergy and Infectious Diseases to involve community physicians in "protocol development and implementation" and to provide direct grant funding "to assist community-based trial sponsors to develop and implement clinical trial protocols" (42). In the fall of 1988, the U.S. Congress appropriated resources for a pilot program "to seed community based clinical trial programs around the country"; the American Foundation for AIDS Research (AmFAR)–funded pilot programs the following year (38). At the time of this writing, public funds continue to support community-based clinical research on HIV disease, through the CPCRA (Community Programs for Clinical Research on AIDS)—a network of community-based health-care providers who have integrated scientific research into their primary care activities (43).

Community Mobilization: Public Health Lessons Learned

Three decades of AIDS provide numerous examples of diverse HIV prevention and treatment issues to which the community has responded: the closing of gay bathhouses as a prevention strategy, broadening the AIDS case definition to include female-specific conditions, federal guidelines for reporting HIV infection by name, strategies to decrease perinatal HIV transmission, and efforts to improve access to early HIV diagnosis and care—to name several prominent examples. Early on, responses from various communities of gay white men tended to predominate, but with the shifting of the epidemic to involve a greater proportion of racial and ethnic minorities and women, so, too, did the community voices involved in mobilization efforts diversify.

What have we learned about community mobilization from our cumulative experience with HIV/AIDS? How can these lessons be applied to help identify and solve other health problems? The most obvious lesson is evident from the preceding discussion: namely, that it isn't always public health and medical leaders who mobilize communities to take appropriate health action. Sometimes communities themselves must mobilize public health and medical leaders to take necessary health actions. The experience of HIV/AIDS is replete with examples of community groups and advocates for PLWHAs pushing forward prevention, medical care, and research agendas. In fact, the success of AIDS activism in the United States has been so compelling that it has been credited as an important influence on the development of patient advocacy groups for other serious illnesses, including breast cancer (31) and Alzheimer's disease (36).

Coalitions have been mobilized to address a wide range of public health problems unrelated to HIV/AIDS, including tobacco control, substance abuse, teen pregnancy, and breast and cervical cancer control (44). Nevertheless, two aspects of community mobilization related to HIV/AIDS are pre-eminent and, by virtue of their conspicuousness, will likely influence future efforts to mobilize communities for health action: enhancing government's ability to understand and work with marginalized populations and increasing community participation in research decision making.

In the early 1990s, directors of fourteen local health departments were surveyed about their perceptions of critical events shaping public health performance during the past decade (45). Out of a list of twenty critical events, including "block grant financing," "loss of federal grants," "local economy," and "change in local political leadership," the HIV/AIDS epidemic was rated as having had the strongest positive impact on the three core public health functions of assessment, policy development, and assurance (45). Positive consequences of the epidemic noted by the respondents included an "increased knowledge of various populations within the community and strengthening of community relationships" (45).

It would be foolhardy to imply that there have been no other variables (beyond HIV/AIDS) influencing a closer collaboration between government and community in the pursuit of shared health goals. Consider that three years before the first reported U.S. AIDS cases the International Conference on Primary Health-care produced the seminal "Alma-Ata Declaration," calling for "maximum community participation in the planning, organization, operation, and control of primary health-care" (46). Moreover, an awareness that health promotion was broader than personal behavior change and individual responsibility burgeoned in the 1980s and shaped an "alternative vision" of health promotion (47)—one predicated on the notion that healthy outcomes could not be achieved without the close cooperation and involvement of affected communities. Although there is no precise way to quantify the discrete contribution of the HIV/AIDS epidemic to governments' ability to better understand and address the public health needs of marginalized and vulnerable populations, it has undoubtedly increased communication between government and affected communities. In the words of Altman, "in a short period of time community organizations, largely representing groups that had previously been somewhat marginalized, have obtained extraordinary legitimacy and access" (48).

In part, improved communications between communities at risk for HIV/AIDS and organized public health is a function of time and experience. Providing federal and state resources to incorporate community-based and other nongovernmental organizations into the delivery system for HIV prevention and care services dates back to the early years of the epidemic in the United States (8,49,50). And, over time, the level of public resources supporting HIV/AIDS activities in non-governmental organizations has increased substantially, thus increasing the frequency and diversity of interactions between governmental and non-governmental organizations involved in these activities. How does this experience inform other aspects of public health? Consider that many of the core competencies deemed necessary for the public health workforce to possess in order to "mobilize community partnerships to identify and solve problems" (51) are the same competencies required to work successfully with HIV/AIDS community advocates and their organizations. These include skills such as interacting sensitively with persons from diverse backgrounds; developing and adapting approaches to problems that take into account cultural differences; establishing ties with nontraditional health-care providers; and fostering community empowerment, involvement, and power sharing (51).

Indirect evidence supporting the assertion that public health competencies in this arena have expanded as a result of the HIV/AIDS experience is provided by Robins and Backstrom (52). When they surveyed state health departments and AIDS community-based organizations (CBOs) in the mid-1990s, they found that "in most states, the relationship between state health departments and the leading AIDS CBOs is, from both parties' perspectives, quite amicable and cooperative" (52). Realizing that these findings were at odds with the common perception that NGO/GO relationships are characterized by conflict, the authors posited that both CBOs and health departments had, over time, developed "greater finesse" in their dealings with each other—an example of familiarity breeding capacity.

Certainly, not all aspects of government and community interaction are perceived as positive, from either perspective (53,54). Nor is this discussion meant to suggest a panacea, conjure stereotypes (e.g., government is incompetent, community is all-knowing), or minimize the inevitable complexities that ensue as a consequence of broadening the circle of entities involved in public health decision making about HIV programs and policies. Nevertheless, in terms of public health practice, strengthening government's ability to understand and work with marginalized populations has improved prevention capacity by expanding both workforce and organizational capacity, two of the three basic elements of public health infrastructure (55). As expressed by McGuire, "consumer participation in the planning, development, and monitoring of HIV/AIDS programs has enriched service delivery"—stimulating, if not demanding, responsiveness, innovation, and accountability from public health (29).

Community Participation in Research Decision Making

Like many other examples given in this text, participatory research did not begin with HIV/AIDS. As chronicled by Coombe in her discussion of "empowerment evaluation," a number of "research traditions" aimed at legitimizing and empowering the role of community members in research predate HIV/AIDS (56). In 1946, Kurt Lewin, "frustrated by the limitations of traditional social science research methods for understanding and addressing complex human problems" (57), espoused "action research" that stressed the active involvement of those affected by the problem in the actual research (58). But holding with the previously stated premise that the tremendous sense of urgency and threat spawned by AIDS resulted in a qualitatively higher level of community response, it is argued that increased community participation in research decision making is another major legacy of HIV/AIDS in the domain of community mobilization.

Clearly, there is no way to quantify the discrete contribution of the HIV/AIDS epidemic to strengthening community participation in research. But we offer evidence of its influence by citing notable examples of participatory HIV/AIDS research, including "grassroots" community trials of aerosolized pentamidine for PCP (38,39,40,59), active involvement of community advisors in the earliest clinical trials of antiretroviral agents (60), and models for bringing community service providers into the domain of HIV prevention research, where they have helped to direct, develop, and evaluate research efforts (61).

In the domain of policy-making related to research on HIV/AIDS, community responses have been singularly instrumental. Pressure from HIV/AIDS community activists has helped to increase AIDS research funding (31,59) and to broaden participation in clinical trials of anti-HIV agents to include women, people of color, drug users, and those with low incomes (30,59). Moreover, legislation responsible for the reorganization of federal HIV/AIDS research efforts in the United States in the early 1990s "owed a great deal" to pressure from HIV/AIDS community advocacy organizations (59). The Office of AIDS Research (OAR), established by the National Institutes of Health (NIH) Revitalization Act of 1993, is responsible for the scientific, budgetary, legislative, and policy elements of the entire HIV research agenda at the NIH; in reaching these critical policy decisions, OAR is mandated to use an advisory council composed of nongovernmental scientific experts and AIDS community representatives (62).

At the onset of the HIV/AIDS era, public health research generally tended to stress individual rather than social risk factors (63). In this it was heavily influenced by biomedical approaches to disease control (64) and cognitive and decision-making theories of human behavior (8). Yet concurrent developments like the 1978 Alma-Ata Declaration on Primary Health-care (46) and the 1986 Ottawa Charter for Health Promotion (65) were helping to advance the notion that health was much more than absence of disease—namely, that "political, economic, social, cultural, environmental, behavioral, and biological factors can all favor health or be harmful to it" (65). Confronted by a disease of unknown etiology that was closely associated with highly stigmatized behaviors, practices, and populations, researchers were unable to avoid or ignore the community context of AIDS. Then, too, the fact that New York City and San Francisco, early American epicenters of the AIDS epidemic, both had strong and visible gay communities (66) helped ensure that scientists studying this new disease couldn't do so without the support and cooperation of gay community leaders. Leaders who consistently challenged the notion of being passive research subjects instead now demanded a role in research decision-making (22,29,59,67).

Contribution of HIV/AIDS to Health Planning

While planning has neither the cachet of investigating a disease outbreak nor the immediate gratification of delivering needed preventive services, it is nevertheless an essential function of public health and a requisite for programs to have successful outcomes. But for a number of reasons, public health agencies may not consistently give adequate attention to accomplishing the planning task (68,69). One reason, as noted by Green, is that "the record of planning is often not good. . . . Plans may fail to be implemented . . . may be implemented and fail to respond adequately to the real needs of the population" (70). Sadly, along with these missteps, planning may come to be erroneously viewed as an end in itself, thus generating cynicism and a consequent reluctance to support necessary planning efforts (70).

Technical complexities, too, can be impediments to health planning. Given that "public health agencies . . . never have adequate resources to address the needs of all constituents" (71), allocative planning (i.e., determining how resources should be spent) is an extremely important dimension of public health planning. But, as noted by Murray, scientific priority setting techniques are constrained by a number of circumstances, including limitations in the available data; choices that cannot be empirically resolved (e.g., how do planners define "health" or reconcile immediate versus longer term health needs, such as investment in risk reduction counseling versus vaccine research); and local variations in health problems and resources (72). Further, priority setting is not purely a function of cost–benefit analysis (73); other principles and values are involved. Three fundamental principles of justice in health-care rationing are highly relevant to decisions about allocating scarce public health resources: need principles (i.e., distribute resources in relation to need), maximizing principles (i.e., distribute resources to achieve maximum health benefit), and egalitarian principles (i.e., distribute resources to reduce inequalities in health) (74). Although it is obvious from the foregoing, it must be stated that there is no single or simple approach to setting priorities during the public health planning process.

HIV Prevention Community Planning

One innovation in allocative public health planning that emerged from the HIV/AIDS experience in the United States has been community planning for HIV prevention (75,76). This nationwide process, first implemented in 1994, requires every health department receiving federal HIV prevention funds to employ a scientifically sound, community-based process to determine the allocation of these funds (77).

HIV prevention community planning strives to ensure that publicly funded HIV prevention programs are based on sound epidemiologic and behavioral science, targeted to those groups at highest risk of acquiring or transmitting HIV infection, and reflective of the needs and preferences of the affected communities for whom they are intended (76). Using data from a variety of sources (e.g., prevention needs assessments, HIV/AIDS surveillance data, behavioral surveys of high risk populations), community planning groups are charged with identifying one or more specific prevention approaches for priority target populations, based on the unique needs and circumstances of their local HIV epidemics. To ensure that resource allocations match the priorities of the plan, planning groups must review and sign off on the states' federal funding applications. As the federal funding entity, the Centers for Disease Control and Prevention is responsible for ensuring that state funding requests do not deviate from plans—or, if they do, that there are appropriate and rational justifications for such deviation (77).

Like most innovations, HIV prevention community planning did not arise de novo. Instead, it grew out of a number of important antecedents (75,78,79,80), including the Centers for Disease Control and Prevention's (CDC) "Planned Approach to Community Health" (PATCH) program, an earlier effort to strengthen health departments' capacity to develop and evaluate health promotion activities directed toward high-priority health problems (81). However, a unique feature of HIV prevention community planning is the substantial budget over which it holds sway—some $300 million federal dollars in 2001. Also distinctive is the planning model's explicit identification of six criteria that must be used when prioritizing HIV prevention strategies and interventions: current and projected need; outcome effectiveness; cost effectiveness; theoretical basis; values, norms, and preferences of the intended audience; and availability of other resources to support the proposed activity (82).

National analyses of health department funding patterns have demonstrated that following the implementation of HIV prevention community planning, the proportion of federal HIV prevention resources supporting health education and risk-reduction activities carried out extramurally (i.e., services provided by local health departments and non-governmental organizations, through subcontract) has increased (83,84). This finding is highly significant given that an overemphasis on clinic-based HIV counseling and testing services was a major criticism of health department prevention programs before HIV prevention community planning. Holtgrave and his colleagues, analyzing community planning groups' allocation of federal resources for health education and risk-reduction activities and HIV counseling and testing, demonstrated improvements between 1997 and 1998 in the racial and ethnic congruity between allocated resources and the burden of HIV infection, as reflected by AIDS prevalence (85).

Lessons Learned from Community Planning for HIV Prevention

In the words of Marmor and Morone, who were analyzing another national effort to improve U.S. health planning (i.e., the National Health Planning and Resources Development Act of 1974), "when plans are isolated from the process of resource allocation and, more generally, from authority—planning can become a smokescreen, a symbol, or simply frustrated wheelspinning" (86). A major objective of HIV prevention community planning is to strengthen the connection between planning, priority setting, and resource allocation, so that funded HIV prevention activities are scientifically sound, targeted to those groups at highest risk of HIV acquisition or transmission, and perceived to be credible by their intended audiences (76).

That HIV prevention community planning has broadened our experience with community participation (see Chapter 8 in this volume) and deepened our understanding of allocative public health planning on a national scale is undeniable (82,83,84,85,87,88,89,90). This is not to say that the process has successfully surmounted all of the barriers that arise when making multilayered funding decisions across a variety of populations and circumstances.

Academicians have noted the inherent difficulties in planning groups' attempts to use cost-effectiveness analyses (91) or to conceptualize specific prevention activities in economic terms of the number of HIV infections averted (92). Practitioners of the planning process complain about the labor intensiveness of HIV prevention community planning (93), cite the complexity of setting priorities (93), and identify a number of barriers to using cost-effectiveness data in "real world" public health decision making. The latter include gaps in available data, lack of "in-house" scientific expertise to help translate and operationalize scientific findings, and conflicts of interest among planning group members (94). And various at-risk communities, particularly racial and ethnic minorities, noting that they are underrepresented on HIV prevention planning groups, question the validity of the planning process (95,96,97).

Many of the concerns raised by participants of HIV prevention community planning have been echoed by those involved in the other major HIV/AIDS planning process in the United States: planning for HIV-related treatment and care funded by the Ryan White Care Act (see Chapter 6 in this volume). Ongoing experiences with Title I (emergency relief grants to designated metropolitan areas) planning councils and Title II (formula grants to states) consortia have also advanced our knowledge base regarding the complexities of health planning (98, 99,100,101). And although it is quite different in process and outcome from HIV prevention community planning, "Ryan White" planning, too, engenders complaints about labor intensiveness, conflicts of interest, and inadequate representation from marginalized populations—especially the economically disenfranchised (101,102).

Certainly, HIV prevention community planning should not be viewed as the ne plus ultra of allocative planning. Laudable though its goals are, community planning hasn't always achieved its intended outcomes (95,96,97). Nor have analysts concluded their debates over optimal methods of allocating public health resources (103); some believe that "federal and state agencies . . . could make better decisions regarding their investments" in HIV prevention (104). In many ways, the major legacy of HIV/AIDS to public health planning has been its ability to spur the development and testing of a logic-based model for targeting finite public health resources (105). For while all agree on the importance of priority setting in public health, there are blessed few examples of models that have been put into practical operation on a nationwide scale. HIV prevention community planning has provided, and tested, tangible models of data-driven, community-based decision making about health priorities that can be applied to other, emerging health threats in both industrialized and developing world settings.

Conclusion

Governmental and community-based organizations providing public health services will be hard-pressed to achieve success without the backing of the communities for whom these services are intended. Further, without adequate planning, public health services may be poorly developed and inappropriately targeted. And policy, program, and research priorities that are out of step with community health concerns and needs are, by definition, unacceptable. Thus, the rich array of community mobilization, priority setting, and health planning experience gained as a result of our collective efforts to vanquish HIV/AIDS is a boon to other areas of public health.

Without doubt, traditionalists have found it challenging to work with community activists and other experts, such as behavioral and social scientists, whose perspectives often extend beyond accepted and well-worn biomedical approaches to public health. How could it be otherwise? Adding multiple voices, new perspectives, and divergent criteria to discussions of problems for which there are no quick, easy, or single solutions is bound to increase complexity—and tensions. But without the experience of HIV/AIDS, public health's admonitions to "empower communities" and "mobilize partnerships to solve health problems" would have remained platitudes—lofty goals devoid of large-scale, practical experience. AIDS changed all of that, to the ultimate benefit of public health.

References

1. Institute of Medicine: Summary and recommendations. In Institute of Medicine: *The Future of Public Health.* National Academy Press, Washington, D.C., 1988, pp. 1–18.
2. Gostin LJ: Public health law in a new century: Part I. Law as a tool to advance the community's health. *JAMA* 283: 2837–2841, 2000.
3. Gostin LJ: Public health law in a new century: Part II. Public health powers and limits. *JAMA* 283: 2979–2984, 2000.
4. Fee E: The origins and development of public health in the United States. In Holland WW, Detels R, and Knox G (eds.): *Oxford Textbook of Public Health.* Oxford University Press, Oxford, 1991, pp. 356–354.
5. Duffy J: Bacteriology revolutionizes public health. In Duffy J: *The Sanitarians: A History of American Public Health.* University of Illinois Press, Urbana, 1990, pp. 193–204.
6. Brandt AM: Damaged goods: progressive medicine and social hygiene. In Brandt AM: *No Magic Bullet: A Social History of Venereal Disease in the United States since 1880.* Oxford University Press, New York, 1985, pp. 7–51.
7. Carlaw RW, Mittlemark MB, Bracht N, and Luepker R: Organization for a community cardiovascular health program: experiences from the Minnesota Heart Health Program. *Health Educ Quart* 11: 243–252, 1984.

8. Valdiserri RO, West GR, Moore M, Darrow WW, and Hinman AR: Structuring HIV prevention service delivery systems on the basis of social science theory. *J Community Health* 17: 259–269, 1992.

9. Freudenberg N and Trinidad U: The role of community organizations in AIDS prevention in two Latino communities in New York City. *Health Educ Quart* 19: 219–232, 1992.

10. Marconi K, Rundall T, Gentry D, Kwait J, Celentano D, and Stolley P: The organization and availability of HIV-related services in Baltimore, Maryland and Oakland, California. *AIDS Public Policy* 9: 173–181, 1994.

11. Joint United Nations Programme on HIV/AIDS: *UNAIDS and Nongovernmental Organizations* (UNAIDS/99.26E). United Nations, Geneva, 1999.

12. Core Functions Project, U.S. Public Health Service: Health-care reform and public health: a paper on population-based core functions. *J Public Health Policy* 19: 394–419, 1998.

13. Lee P and Paxman D: Reinventing public health. *Annu Rev Public Health* 18: 1–35, 1997.

14. Trevino FM and Jacobs JP: Public health and health-care reform: the American Public Health Association's perspective. *J Public Health Policy* 15: 397–406, 1994.

15. Centers for Disease Control and Prevention: Public opinion about public health—United States, 1999. *Morb Mortal Wkly Rep* 49: 258–260, 2000.

16. Centers for Disease Control and Prevention: Public opinion about public health—California and the United States, 1996. *Morb Mortal Wkly Rep* 47: 69–73, 1998.

17. Heffler S, Levit K, Smith S, Smith C, Cowan C, Lazenby H, and Freeland M: Health spending growth up in 1999: faster growth expected in the future. *Health Affairs* 20: 193–203, 2001.

18. Eilbert KW, Barry M, Bialek R, Garufi M, Maiese D, Gebbie K, and Fox CE: Public health expenditures: developing estimates for improved policy making. *J Public Health Manag Pract* 3: 1–9, 1997

19. Freudenberg N and Zimmerman MA: The role of community organizations in public health practice: the lessons from AIDS prevention. In Freudenberg N and Zimmerman MA (eds.): *AIDS Prevention in the Community.* American Public Health Association, Washington, DC, 1995, pp. 183–197.

20. Minkler M: Introduction and overview. In Minkler M (ed.): *Community Organizing and Community Building for Health.* Rutgers University Press, New Brunswick, NJ, 1997, pp. 3–19.

21. Minkler M and Wallerstein N: Improving health through community organization and community building: a health education perspective. In Minkler M (ed.): *Community Organizing and Community Building for Health.* Rutgers University Press, New Brunswick, NJ, 1997, pp. 30–52.

22. Bastos C: Politics and the construction of knowledge. In Bastos C: *Global Responses to AIDS: Science in Emergency.* Indiana University Press, Bloomington, 1999, pp. 23–49.

23. Andriote J: In memoriam. In Andriote J: *Victory Deferred: How AIDS Changed Gay Life in America.* University of Chicago Press, Chicago, 1999, pp. 331–369.

24. Centers for Disease Control and Prevention: Update: acquired immunodeficiency syndrome in the San Francisco cohort study, 1978–1985. *Morb Mortal Wkly Rep* 34: 573–575, 1985.

25. UNAIDS/WHO Working Group on Global HIV/AIDS and STI Surveillance: *Botswana: Epidemiological Fact Sheet on HIV/AIDS and Sexually Transmitted Infections.* World Health Organization, Geneva, 2000, p. 3.

26. Institute of Medicine: Summary and Recommendations. In Institute of Medicine: *Confronting AIDS: Direction for Public Health, Health-Care, and Research.* National Academy Press, Washington, DC, 1986, pp. 5–35.

27. Panem S: Economics and politics. In Panem S: *The AIDS Bureaucracy: Why Society Failed to Meet the AIDS Crisis and How We Might Improve our Response.* Harvard University Press, Cambridge, MA, 1988, pp. 72–85.

28. Christoffel KK: Public health advocacy: process and product. *Am J Public Health* 90: 722–726, 2000.

29. McGuire J: Inclusion, representation, and parity: the making of a public health response to HIV. In Mayer KH and Pizer HF (eds.): *The Emergence of AIDS: The Impact on Immunology, Microbiology, and Public Health.* American Public Health Association, Washington, DC, 2000, pp. 181–205.

30. Fee E and Krieger N: Understanding AIDS: historical interpretations and the limits of biomedical individualism. *Am J Public Health* 83: 1477–1486, 1993.

31. Wachter RM: AIDS, activism, and the politics of health. *N Engl J Med* 326: 128–132, 1992.

32. Andriote J: Introduction. In Andriote J: *Victory Deferred: How AIDS Changed Gay Life in America.* University of Chicago Press, Chicago, 1999, pp. 1–5.

33. Wolfred TR: Ending the HIV epidemic: a call for community action. In Petrow S, Franks P, and Wolfred TR (eds.): *Ending the HIV Epidemic: Community Strategies in Disease Prevention and Health Promotion.* Network Publications, Santa Cruz, CA, 1990, pp. 132–139.

34. Brown, J (ed.): *A Promise to Remember: The Names Project Book of Letters.* Avon Books, New York, 1992.

35. Fabj V and Sobnosky MJ: Responses from the street: ACT UP and community organizing against AIDS. In Ratzan SC (ed.): *AIDS: Effective Health Communication for the 90s.* Taylor and Francis, Washington, DC, 1993, pp. 91–109.

36. Edgar H and Rothman D: New rules for new drugs: the challenge of AIDS to the regulatory process. *Millbank Quart* 68: 111–142, 1990.

37. James JS: Update: community-based trials and San Francisco's Community Research Alliance. *AIDS Treatment News* 85(August 11, 1989): 1–7.

38. Harrington M: The Community Research Initiative (CRI) of New York: clinical research and prevention treatments. In Van Vugt JP (ed.): *AIDS Prevention and Services: Community Based Research.* Bergin and Garvey, Westport, CT, 1994, pp. 153–178.

39. Sonnabend J, Blau A, Freeman K, Holzemer S, and Forrest J: Aerosolized pentamidine (AP) improves diffusion capacity in AIDS patients with no history of *P. carinii* pneumonia (PCP) (#W.B. 2187). Paper presented at the Seventh International Conference on AIDS, Florence, June 16–21, 1991.

40. Leoung GS, Feigal DW, Montgomery B, Corkery K, Wardlaw L, Adams M, Busch D, Gordon S, Jacobson MA, Volberding PA, and Abrams D: Aerosolized pentamidine for prophylaxis against *Pneumocystis carinii* pneumonia: the San Francisco Community Prophylaxis Trial. *N Engl J Med* 323: 769–775, 1990.

41. Centers for Disease Control and Prevention: Guidelines for prophylaxis against *Pneumocystis carinii* pneumonia for persons infected with human immunodeficiency virus. *Morb Mortal Wkly Rep* 38: 1–9, 1989.

42. Presidential Commission on the Human Immunodeficiency Virus: *Report to the President of the United States.* U.S. Govt. Printing Office, Washington, DC, 1988, p. 58.

43. Community Programs for Clinical Research on AIDS: Research studies. URL: www.cpcra.org/res-studies.htm (December 2001).

44. Kegler MC, Steckler A, McLeroy K, and Malek SH: Factors that contribute to effective community health promotion coalitions: a study of 10 Project ASSIST coalitions in North Carolina. *Health Educ Behav* 25: 338–353, 1998.

45. Miller CA, Moore KS, and Richards TB: The impact of critical events of the 1980s on core functions for a selected group of local health departments. *Public Health Rep* 108: 695–700, 1993.

46. World Health Organization: Declaration of Alma-Ata: International Conference on Primary Health-care, Alma-Ata, USSR, 6–12 September 1978. URL: www.who.dk/policy/almaata.htm.

47. Minkler M: Health education, health promotion and the open society: an historical perspective. *Health Educ Quart* 16: 17–30, 1989.

48. Altman D: The evolution of the community sector. In Altman D: *Power and Community: Organizational and Cultural Responses to AIDS.* Taylor and Francis, London, 1994, pp. 97–117.

49. Bailey M: Community-based organizations and CDC as partners in HIV education and prevention. *Public Health Rep* 106: 702–708, 1991.

50. Holman PB, Jenkins WC, Gayle JA, Duncan C, and Lindsey BK: Increasing the involvement of national and regional racial and ethnic minority organizations in HIV information and education. *Public Health Rep* 106: 687–694, 1991.

51. Public Health Functions Project: *The Public Health Workforce: An Agenda for the 21st Century.* Department of Health and Human Services, Washington, DC, 1997, pp. 29–42.

52. Robins L and Backstrom C: Organizational imperatives and policy perspectives of AIDS community-based organizations: a view from the states. *AIDS Public Policy* 14: 3–19, 1999.

53. Cain R: Community-based AIDS organizations and the state: dilemmas of dependence. *AIDS Public Policy* 10: 83–93, 1995.

54. Altman D: Change, co-option and the community sector. *AIDS* 9: S239–S243, 1995.

55. Centers for Disease Control and Prevention: *Public Health's Infrastructure: A Status Report.* Centers for Disease Control and Prevention, Atlanta, 2000, pp. 5–6.

56. Coombe CM: Using empowerment evaluation in community organizing and community-based health initiatives. In Minkler M (ed.): *Community Organizing and Community Building for Health.* Rutgers University Press, New Brunswick, NJ, 1997, pp. 291–307.

57. Minkler M: Using participatory action research to build healthy communities. *Public Health Rep* 115: 191–197, 2000.

58. Lewin K: Action research and minority problems. *J Soc Issues* 2: 34–36, 1946.

59. Altman D: The changing pandemic. In Altman D: *Power and Community: Organizational and Cultural Responses to AIDS.* Taylor and Francis, London, 1994, pp. 67–96.

60. Valdiserri RO, Tama GH, and Ho M: The role of community advisory committees in clinical trials of anti-HIV agents. *IRB: Rev Hum Subj Res* 10: 5–7, 1988.

61. Sanstad KH, Stall R, Goldstein E, Everett W, and Brousseau R: Collaborative community research consortium: a model for HIV prevention. *Health Educ Behav* 26: 171–184, 1999.

62. About OAR. URL: www.nih.gov/od/oar (September 2000).

63. Israel BA, Schulz AJ, and Parker EA: Review of community-based research: assessing partnership approaches to improve public health. *Annu Rev Public Health* 19: 173–202, 1998.

64. Valdiserri RO: Historical variables influencing AIDS prevention programs. In Valdiserri RO: *Preventing AIDS: The Design of Effective Programs.* Rutgers University Press, New Brunswick, NJ, 1989, pp. 24–41.

65. World Health Organization: Ottawa Charter for Health Promotion: First International Conference on Health Promotion, Ottawa, Canada, November 17–21, 1986. URL: www.who.dk/policy/ottawa.htm.

66. Andriote J: The field. In Andriote J: *Victory Deferred: How AIDS Changed Gay Life in America.* University of Chicago Press, Chicago, 1999, pp. 7–45.

67. Harden VA and Rodrigues D: Context for a new disease: aspects of biomedical research policy in the United States before AIDS. In Berridge V and Strong P (eds.): *AIDS and Contemporary History.* Cambridge University Press, Cambridge, 1993, pp. 182–202.

68. Steuart G: The importance of programme planning. *Health Educ Quart* S1: S21–S27, 1993.

69. Institute of Medicine: An assessment of the current public health system: a shattered vision. In Institute of Medicine: *The Future of Public Health.* National Academy Press, Washington, DC, 1988, pp. 73–106.

70. Green A: What is planning, and why plan? In Green A: *An Introduction to Health Planning in Developing Countries,* 2nd ed. Oxford University Press, Oxford, 1999, pp. 1–23.

71. Vilnius D and Dandoy S: A priority rating system for public health programs. *Public Health Rep* 105: 463–470, 1990.

72. Murray CJL: Rational approaches to priority setting in international health. *Am J Trop Med Hyg* 93: 303–311, 1990.

73. Bosin MR: Priority setting in government: beyond the magic bullet. *Eval Program Plann* 15: 33–43, 1992.

74. Cookson R and Dolan P: Principles of justice in health care rationing. *J Med Ethics* 26: 323–329, 2000.

75. Valdiserri RO, Aultman TV, and Curran JW: Community planning: a national strategy to improve HIV prevention programs. *J Community Health* 20: 87–100, 1995.

76. Valdiserri RO: Managing system-wide change in HIV prevention programs: a CDC perspective. *Public Admin Rev* 56: 545–553, 1996.

77. Centers for Disease Control and Prevention: *Supplemental Guidance on HIV Prevention Community Planning for Noncompeting Continuation of Cooperative Agreements for HIV Prevention Projects.* CDC, Atlanta, 1993.

78. State Health Agency Vision Working Group: *State Health Agency Vision for HIV Prevention.* Association of State and Territorial Health Officials, National Alliance of State and Territorial AIDS Directors, and Council of State and Territorial Epidemiologists, Washington DC, 1993.

79. Valdiserri RO and West GR: Barriers to the assessment of unmet need in planning HIV/AIDS prevention programs. *Public Admin Rev* 54: 25–30, 1994.

80. Schietinger H, Coburn J, and Levi J: Community planning for HIV prevention: findings from the first year. *AIDS Public Policy* 10: 140–147, 1995.

81. Kreuter MW: PATCH: its origin, basic concepts, and links to contemporary public health policy. *J Health Educ* 23: 135–139, 1992.

82. Pinkerton SD, Holtgrave DR, Willingham M, and Goldstein E: Cost-effectiveness analysis and HIV prevention community planning. *AIDS Public Policy* 13: 115–127, 1998.

83. Valdiserri RO, Robinson C, Lin LS, West GR, and Holtgrave DR: Determining al-

locations for HIV-prevention interventions: assessing a change in federal funding policy. *AIDS Public Policy* 12: 138–148, 1997.

84. Renaud M and Kresse E: *HIV Prevention Community Planning Profiles: Assessing the Impact.* United States Conference of Mayors, Washington DC, 1996, pp. 87–94.

85. Holtgrave DR, Thomas CW, Chen H, Edlavitch S, Pinkerton SD, and Fleming P: HIV prevention community planning and communities of color: do resources track the epidemic? *AIDS Public Policy* 15: 75–81, 2000.

86. Marmor TR and Morone JA: Representing consumer interests: imbalanced markets, health planning, and the HSAs. *Milbank Mem Fund Quart* 58: 125–165, 1980.

87. Holtgrave DR and Valdiserri RO: Year one HIV prevention community planning: a national perspective on accomplishments, challenges, and future directions. *J Public Health Manag Pract* 2: 1–9, 1996.

88. Dearing JW, Larson RS, Randall LM, and Pope RS: Local reinvention of the CDC HIV prevention community planning initiative. *J Community Health* 23: 113–126, 1998.

89. Cotten-Oldenburg NU, Rosser BRS, DeBoer J, Rugg DL, and Carr P: Building strong linkages across the HIV prevention continuum: the practical lessons learned from a comprehensive evaluation effort in Minnesota. *AIDS Educ Prev* 13: 29–41, 2001.

90. Roe KM, Berenstein C, Goette C, and Roe K: Community building through empowering evaluation: a case study of HIV prevention community planning. In Minkler M (ed.): *Community Organizing and Community Building for Health.* Rutgers University Press, New Brunswick, NJ, 1997, pp. 308–322.

91. Kahn JG and Haynes-Sanstad KC: The role of cost-effectiveness analysis in assessing HIV-prevention interventions. *AIDS Public Policy* 12: 21–30, 1997.

92. Kaplan EH: Economic evaluation and HIV prevention community planning: a policy analyst's perspective. In Holtgrave DR (ed.): *Handbook of Economic Evaluation of HIV Prevention Programs.* Plenum Press, New York, 1998, pp. 177–193.

93. National Alliance of State and Territorial AIDS Directors: *HIV Prevention Community Planning: Co-chairs' Perspectives.* Washington, DC, 1999, pp. 1–20.

94. Weinstein B and Melchreit RL: Economic evaluation and HIV prevention decision making: the state perspective. In Holtgrave DR (ed.): *Handbook of Economic Evaluation of HIV Prevention Programs.* Plenum Press, New York, 1998, pp. 153–162.

95. Maldonado M: *HIV/AIDS and African Americans.* National Minority AIDS Council, Washington, DC, 1999, pp. 1–13.

96. Maldonado M: *HIV/AIDS and Latinos.* National Minority AIDS Council, Washington, DC, 1999, pp. 1–14.

97. Bau I: Asians and Pacific Islanders and HIV prevention community planning. *AIDS Educ Prev* 10(Suppl. A): 77–93, 1998.

98. United States General Accounting Office: *Use of Ryan White CARE Act and Other Assistance Grant Funds.* U.S. General Accounting Office, Washington, DC, 2000, pp. 1–51.

99. Kachur S, Sonnega AJ, Cintron R, Farup C, Silbersiepe K, Celentano DD, and Kwait J: An analysis of the Greater Baltimore HIV services planning council. *AIDS Public Policy* 7: 238–246, 1992.

100. Buchanan RJ: HIV consortia services funded by Title II of the Ryan White CARE Act: a survey of the states. *AIDS Public Policy* 11: 118–143, 1996.

101. Bradford J, Honnold J, Rives ME, and Hafford K: The effectiveness of resource allocation methods used by RWCA Title II consortia in Virginia. *AIDS Public Policy* 15: 29–42, 2000.

102. Bowen GS, Marconi K, Kohn S, Bailey DM, Goosby EP, Shorter S, and Niemcryk, S: First year of AIDS services delivery under Title I of the Ryan White CARE Act. *Public Health Rep* 107: 491–499, 1992.
103. Catania JA, Morin SF, Canchola J, Pollack L, Chang J, and Coates TJ: U.S. priorities—HIV prevention. *Science* 290: 717, 2000.
104. Committee on HIV Prevention Strategies in the United States: *No Time to Lose: Getting More from HIV Prevention.* National Academy Press, Washington, DC, 2001.
105. Johnson-Masotti AP, Pinkerton SD, and Holtgrave DR: Prioritization methods for community planning. *J Public Health Manag Pract* 6: 72–85, 2000.

4

Innovations in Approaches to Preventing HIV/AIDS: Applications to Other Health Promotion Activities

ANN O'LEARY, DAVID R. HOLTGRAVE,
LINDA WRIGHT-DeAQÜERO, AND ROBERT M. MALOW

In 1983, public health researchers unveiled the first study showing that the acquired immune deficiency syndrome (AIDS) is transmitted by sexual behavior (1,2). Not long afterward, it was learned that HIV is also transmitted by injection drug use (3). Therefore, early HIV prevention efforts, conducted by community organizations like San Francisco's "Stop AIDS" and New York's "Gay Men's Health Crisis," encouraged people to refrain from sexual and drug use activities that placed them at risk of infection. To the extent that sexual abstinence was not possible, the use of male, latex condoms was encouraged. To the extent that abstinence from drug injection was not possible, the use of bleach to disinfect injection equipment was encouraged. Over time, rigorously evaluated interventions to promote sexual risk reduction (4) and injection drug use (5) added to a growing portfolio of HIV risk-reduction interventions that were founded primarily on basic principles of behavior change. Research activities throughout the first two decades of the AIDS epidemic were deemed highly successful in identifying efficacious and effective intervention models (6).

HIV prevention research has focused concern on the subtleties of an unusually broad array of risk factors, such as substance abuse and addiction, limited empowerment of women, male resistance to using condoms, traditional socialized sex roles, adolescent development issues, past and current physical and sexual abuse, psychiatric co-morbidities, and life problems associated with poverty and inner-city living. More recently, assessments of the state-of-the-art in HIV risk reduction (7–10) have highlighted the importance of so-called background or contextual factors as pivotal determinants of intervention outcomes. Although the appreciation of contextual factors is certainly not new to understanding infectious disease risk, it would be difficult to name another illness or condition in which researchers have so consistently attended to the underlying context of risk in the development of interventions. Namely, in developing and testing interventions, behavioral and social scientists have considered the overlapping role that psychosocial, physical, political, and economic environments play in mediating risk behavior and responses to risk.

Fueled by the intense focus on contextual factors, there is a rapidly expanding emphasis on identifying, developing, and testing structural interventions to reduce HIV risk (11). Structural interventions are those that attempt to directly or indirectly influence HIV transmission by modifying laws, regulations, policies, systems, and/or environmental factors. This interest in structural factors represents a further recognition that behavior change approaches alone are not enough to halt HIV transmission, and without a supportive policy environment, behavioral interventions may be doomed to failure (12).

Implementing HIV risk-reduction interventions has met with numerous challenges. These challenges have included (*a*) the need to custom tailor the interventions to those most likely to be affected—marginalized, stigmatized, and impoverished populations; (*b*) the critical need to integrate HIV prevention with other key social and health services; (*c*) the fact that drug use and sex are highly reinforcing, potentially addictive, activities that are difficult to modify; (*d*) the need to recognize that HIV-related behaviors occur in dyads and groups (requiring programs to intervene at those social levels); (*e*) the difficulty of achieving and sustaining large-scale translations of effective, research-based interventions into HIV prevention programs; and (*f*) policy barriers to the delivery of effective interventions. We do not argue that these issues are entirely unique to HIV or AIDS, but the availability of curative treatment for several other sexually transmitted diseases may lessen the need to address these challenges in that domain. In this chapter, we make the case that the approaches to meeting these challenges have provided some of the most interesting lessons in HIV prevention, with import for other areas in public health beyond HIV prevention.

Effects on Marginalized Populations

HIV/AIDS has disproportionately affected racial, ethnic and sexual minorities in the United States. It is estimated that people of color account for over half of new HIV infections annually (13); men who have sex with men account for an estimated 42 percent of incident HIV infection, and injection drug users for an estimated 25 percent of annual infections. Women now account for approximately

30 percent of new HIV infections. The percentage of AIDS cases among women was 7 percent in 1985 and increased to 23 percent by 1999 (14).

Many of these same groups suffer from disproportionate effects of other diseases, heightened levels of poverty and unemployment, and diminished access to quality health-care services (15). This disenfranchisement may foster, and in turn is fostered by, substance use and trading of sex for drugs or money. In fact, these practices have led some to question whether HIV prevention efforts, by themselves, can do any good unless the fundamental social conditions are first addressed; others believe that both HIV and unhealthy social conditions can be addressed at the same time (16).

The fact that HIV so disproportionately affects the poor and disenfranchised has influenced many aspects of behavioral interventions. For example, many risk-reduction interventions are delivered in settings where high-risk behavior is taking place or other related risks are addressed. These include low-income public housing projects (17), correctional facilities (18,19), street-level interventions (20), public clinics treating sexually transmitted diseases (21), and drug treatment programs (22).

Second, to enhance access to affected communities, several large-scale trials have recruited and trained community members to deliver and reinforce theory-based prevention materials and messages to their peers. For example, the AIDS Community Demonstration Project (23) provided outreach to sex workers, gay men, and men who have sex with men who are not gay-identified. The National AIDS Demonstration Research provided outreach to injection drug users and their sex partners (24,25). Kelly and colleagues (26) used peer outreach to gay men in gay bars. One of the most important contributions of these studies was to demonstrate that theory-based interventions and behavioral assessments could be delivered by trained indigenous outreach workers (27).

This focus on outreach to provide public health services has expanded beyond the HIV arena to other public health areas. For example, a recent study reached low-income teens for nutrition counseling through public housing developments (28), and immunization has also been provided in this setting (29). Likewise, health promotion in correctional facilities has greatly expanded in recent years (30). While it is difficult to argue conclusively that the HIV prevention experience played a causal role in these developments, we believe it likely influenced this expansion.

Populations that are "hidden" due to stigmatization or the wish to remain anonymous have required researchers to tailor their research designs considerably. Roffman and colleagues have used telephone conference calls to provide prevention messages and support to "closeted, rural gay men" (31). Other researchers have asked research participants to recruit additional participants, particularly injection drug users (32,33). Social networks have also been used to deliver interventions. In an adaptation of Rogers's diffusion of innovation theory,

(34) Kelly and colleagues trained popular opinion leaders to give prevention messages to clients in gay bars (26), and this has also been done with women in low-income housing (17). Indeed, diffusion theory has become an important component of community-wide interventions that seek to influence social norms regarding consistent use of condoms and one-time use of sterile syringes. HIV prevention efforts have fostered the broader incorporation of this approach into public health efforts.

Evaluation efforts have also been affected by the desire for anonymity in studies of sensitive behavior. For example, in one study of college students, responses were anonymous, with respondents receiving payment by returning a self-addressed postcard under separate cover from the questionnaire. Researchers preserved the ability to link responses from the same individual over time by creating a "guided code" on the survey that uniquely identified individuals without revealing their identities. Respondents circled letters, numbers, and months corresponding to birthdays, family names, and other personal indicants that are not forgotten and that do not change over time (35). Many of these innovations predated HIV. However, their enhanced use by HIV researchers influenced improvements in their design and their diffusion into other domains of public health.

HIV prevention community planning is another example of an innovation through which the prevention needs of marginalized populations have been given increased and improved attention as a result of the HIV/AIDS experience. Community planning describes the mandated federal process by which state and local health departments must allocate their federal HIV prevention resources. As discussed extensively in Chapter 3 of this volume, HIV prevention community planning was implemented in 1994 to ensure that community voices are heard in the setting of HIV prevention priorities, that HIV prevention resources are allocated in accordance with the trajectories of the epidemic, and that interventions are science based and effective. Community planning provides the mechanism for input on innovative prevention approaches, such as the use of faith communities, outreach to incarcerated populations, use of traditional healers, and involvement of the small business sector (e.g., owners of beauty parlors and bodegas). Because it provides a working model for involving community representatives, along with scientific and technical experts, in public heath decision making and priority setting, it is highly relevant to other public health domains beyond HIV/AIDS.

Co-occurring HIV Risk and Many Other Serious Problems

In the United States, HIV has predominantly affected people who live in a nexus of risk that includes poverty, drug addiction, mental illness, trauma, incarceration, and other severe life stressors (36,37). This is true for the most at-risk groups, including women, injection drug users, and men who have sex with men. While white, often middle-class, gay men were prominently affected early in the epidemic, the gay men currently at risk for HIV infections and AIDS are most frequently men of color, particularly African Americans and Hispanics (38). Substance use is tightly linked to HIV risk among all affected populations. The link with drug use has both direct and indirect elements (39). The direct pathway is the sharing of injection equipment, the reported exposure category of 21 percent of men and 20 percent of women diagnosed with HIV or AIDS during 2000 (13). Indirect causes include sex-for-drug-exchanges (40,41), and, possibly, the psychological effects of drugs and alcohol, leading to lowered concern about personal safety or the safety of others (42,43).

Researchers and service providers are coming to recognize that addressing single issues (e.g., HIV prevention) within the nexus of risk may be ineffective (37,39,44); such thinking may culminate in a revolutionary reconceptualization, even reorganization, of public health research and practice. Consider an early study showing that women with many pressing concerns ranked HIV risk reduction as a relatively low priority (45). Subsequent HIV research has reinforced the notion that coping with problems related to finances, housing, child care, transportation, employment, medical care, maintaining intimate relationships, and personal or neighborhood substance abuse and crime (46–48) may often supersede any efforts to reduce HIV and other health-related risks. In the case of HIV prevention, it has become evident that competing issues actually impede people's ability to change behavior. Drug addiction leads to the exchange of sex for drugs; women experiencing domestic violence are less likely to request that their partners use condoms (48,49). Homelessness can lead to the exchange of sex for shelter or protection. Psychological depression is associated with reduced behavior-change response to sexual risk-reduction counseling (50–52), possibly because it is associated with the use of alcohol and other drugs for self-soothing of distress (53). Even boredom associated with unemployment can contribute to drug use and relapse and to increased sexual activity.

Fundamentally, the fragmentation of public funding streams (i.e., public resources allocated by disease or circumscribed population) impedes progress in addressing the nexus of risk in terms of both service provision and research (54). Community-based organizations can only provide comprehensive services by receiving funding from multiple sources (55). Even health departments receiving funding from multiple sources may experience difficulty in developing comprehensive interventions. HIV specialists are acutely aware of this situation, and examples do exist of interventions targeting the risk nexus. For example, building on the understanding of the multiplicity of needs of youth, some youth interventions have directed their focus to providing educational opportunities, job readiness training, service learning, alternative recreational opportunities, self-esteem building, and education and counseling on the risk of teen sexual activity and substance use (56,57).

Because case management interventions are a model for providing multiple services to individuals, they provide another example of interventions to address multiple risks and needs. Prevention case management for at-risk seronegatives has become an important component of community HIV prevention efforts (58). Case management has been an essential component of HIV primary care even before the advent of highly active antiretroviral therapy. However, recent studies have demonstrated that HIV patients with case managers have fewer unmet needs and higher use of HIV medication (59). Further, HIV primary care case management services are increasingly recognized as important modalities though which to deliver HIV and STD risk-reduction messages and services (58).

Difficulty in Changing Behavior Related to HIV Risk

Sex is quite obviously the behavior most strongly induced by natural selection—the behavior most directly related to reproductive fitness. It is thus (arguably) the most pleasurable of human activities and the most essential for the creation of pair-bonds. Unfortunately, condoms reduce both the pleasure and intimacy that is derived from sex. The impulse to have sex, and to progress toward orgasm once sexually aroused, while of variable intensity and controllability, can often be overpowering. This further reduces the likelihood that the sexual episode will be interrupted to obtain or apply a condom. Similarly, behaviors related to drug use are very difficult to modify. The sharing of drug injection equipment often occurs in connection with drug cravings or withdrawal, social pressure, and, in many places, the unavailability of sterile injection equipment. Once again, the ability to control impulse long enough to reduce the risk of this behavior—for example, by cleaning needles with bleach—is not easily achieved.

Because HIV risk reduction entails particularly difficult behavior change, at-risk individuals often use their own "commonsense" theories of illness (60) to justify making alternative, less-safe changes that are also less difficult. For example, gay men report internally voicing lay beliefs before having unprotected sex that can best be understood as a way to justify the behavior about to be performed (61). These include "HIV is hard to transmit" and "he must be positive himself if he's letting me do this." The tendency of gay men to assume concordant HIV serostatus in a sex partner has also been reported (CDC, Seropositive Urban Men's Study, unpublished data, 2000). Several studies have shown that people adopt "grey-area" behaviors to reduce risk without having to use condoms (62,63). These include withdrawing prior to ejaculation, using serostatus information to determine sexual roles (e.g., during anal sex the seropositive partner is receptive and the seronegative partner is insertive), and using personal algorithms to select partners. That these behaviors are adopted in the absence of scientific establishment of their effectiveness is a testament to the strong aversion that many people have to using condoms.

HIV specialists have grappled with this challenge—that HIV risk behaviors are difficult to change—in several ways. Throughout the epidemic, efforts have been under way to develop an effective preventive vaccine, which might render behavior change unnecessary. In the meantime, some alternatives to condom use have become available. One is joint antibody testing by a couple, which in the case of seroconcordant individuals may be followed by mutual monogamy or at least the agreement to use condoms outside of the primary relationship ("negotiated safety") (64). In fact, a variety of strategies other than condom use may have at least partial effectiveness in preventing HIV (65).

Because of the difficulty in changing HIV risk behaviors, structural interventions have been sought as a means to supplement individual level interventions. Structural interventions are not new to public health. But the HIV/AIDS epidemic has prompted a renewed focus on the importance of laws, regulations, resource allocation, infrastructural development, and system changes that work in concert with individual level interventions to promote behavior change. One notable example is the "100 percent condom use" campaign in Thailand (66). Brothel managers were required to enforce consistent condom use by their sex work staff and clients. Mass media campaigns promoting AIDS awareness and urging condom use occurred simultaneously. During the years when the program was implemented, rates of other STDs dropped dramatically, and HIV prevalence stabilized among the military (2–3 percent) and among pregnant women (1–2 percent). Similar programs were instituted in legalized brothels in Nevada (67). Improvement of the STD control infrastructure to reduce HIV transmission is another example (68). Structural interventions to prevent needle-sharing have centered primarily on the decriminalization of, and increased legal availability of, sterile injection equipment (69). For HIV counseling and testing, publicly funded test sites offering free anonymous or confidential testing were created throughout the United States (70).

Interest in structural interventions in the HIV domain is part of a historical and currently growing interest in structural solutions for numerous other public health problems. Taxation of tobacco and alcohol products is one example; in fact, evidence exists that excise taxation of alcohol affects rates of sexually transmitted disease (71,72), and the CDC has recommended increased taxation of tobacco to discourage tobacco use. Regulations regarding placement of cigarette machines is another example of a structural intervention to limit access to underage smokers. In the violence arena, laws concerning gun sales and technical strategies such as trigger locks are examples of structural interventions. Juvenile curfews are another structural approach to violence (73). Injury prevention relies on structural approaches such as laws for seat belt use, speeding, and drunk driving. Obesity contributes to many health problems; structural approaches such as imposing an excise tax on unhealthy food items such as fast foods, and regulation of the media, have been suggested (74,75). Exercise can be promoted when local communities vote to create bicycle paths and side-walks.

Indeed, the activist movement to promote the structural intervention of mak-ing sterile injection equipment available to injection drug users has promoted the rise of the harm-reduction movement (76). Initially, advocates reasoned that HIV was a much more severe health issue than addiction; their aim was to protect from HIV infection even if drug use could not be discontinued. The concept of "harm reduction" has since evolved to denote any reduction in harm, even par-tial reduction in HIV risk (77).

Harm reduction represents a profoundly important revolution in how public health workers think about risk and harm. It has reduced the "all-or-nothing" thinking that guided medicine for many years. The popularity of the "stages of change" model of behavior change reflects this shift as well, in its implication that movement can occur in increments rather than all at once. Although it is dif-ficult to specify the extent to which HIV efforts have influenced the application of the harm-reduction approach to other areas of public health, examples do ex-ist. The movement in alcohol treatment from an abstinence model to the possi-bility of controlled drinking is one example (78). Harm reduction in smoking has taken the forms of changing tobacco use patterns (e.g., by prohibiting smoking in indoor public spaces); reducing levels of tar, nicotine and pesticides in tobacco; and nicotine replacement (79).

Couples and Group Risk Behavior

The most important risk behaviors for HIV—namely, having unprotected sex and sharing needles—are intrinsically social in nature. However, because most health behavior theories available at the dawn of the epidemic were predicated on in-dividual behavior change (based on smoking cessation, weight control, increased exercise, etc.), they were the first to be deployed in the development of behav-ioral HIV interventions (80). Indeed, to date, the vast majority of behavioral in-terventions that have been evaluated have focused on individuals (81). However, there have been notable exceptions in which couples have been the unit of in-tervention. Roth and colleagues (82) and Coates and colleagues (83) have stud-ied effects of HIV antibody testing on behavior change among couples who have been tested together. Carballo-Dieguez and Remien (84) are currently conduct-ing interventions for HIV-serodiscordant gay men. An intervention for serodis-cordant heterosexual couples is ongoing at the time of this writing (85). How-ever, only one study, currently ongoing, is comparing the effectiveness of interventions delivered to individual women versus to couples. El-Bassel (86) and colleagues are in the follow-up phase of a study in which women were random-ized to receive interventions either with or without the participation of their male partners.

Among injection drug users, the analogous intervention approach would be to deliver an intervention to members of needle-sharing networks. In one study by Latkin and colleagues (33), injection drug users recruited members of their drug-using networks; the intervention was successful in reducing the sharing of needles and other drug paraphernalia.

Interventions in Other Areas of Public Health

Although it is not clear to what extent these interventions were influenced by ongoing HIV prevention experience, or, to what extent they have influenced the development of innovations in HIV prevention interventions, there have clearly been advances in supraindividual interventions directed toward sexual health issues that owe a debt to the HIV/AIDS experience. Miller and colleagues demonstrated the importance of maternal communication on adolescents' subsequent condom use as an example of a behavioral intervention likely to be used in other areas of the health field, especially pregnancy prevention (87). A program of research that has been conducted for several years has intervened with the spouses of patients who suffer from coronary heart disease (88). Spouses are taught to support behavioral changes the patient has been asked to make, such as smoking cessation, dietary changes, and medication compliance. In some studies, wives watched their post-myocardial infarction husbands undergo treadmill evaluations and then took the test themselves, so that their confidence in their husbands' stamina would be boosted and they would be less likely to collude in cardiac invalidism (89). Another public health arena in which both marital partners have participated in interventions is in treatment for drug and alcohol addiction. Here the drug user and spouse make a joint pact each day for the user to stay abstinent. For example, in one study (90), substance-abusing men were randomized to receive individual treatment with or without adjunctive behavioral couple's therapy. Those who received the couple's therapy enhancement reported less drug use and more abstinent days than men receiving individual treatment only. Findings relating social support to diagnostic tests such as mammography (91) have probably influenced current public service announcements calling for womens' friends or family to encourage them to schedule mammograms.

Translation Challenges

HIV prevention interventions have real life-saving potential. However, the translation of interventions found effective in research settings into ongoing HIV prevention programs has met with significant challenges; and the response to these challenges is of relevance to other diseases of public health significance.

Because HIV disease most often affects marginalized, stigmatized, and impoverished communities (especially communities of color), custom-tailoring interventions to the life circumstances, including the cultural context of the community, is likely to be of exceptional importance. Attention to such contextual factors is vital to ensure that efficacious research-based interventions be made both feasible and viable in community settings. As discussed in a recent report from the Institute of Medicine (92), interventions cannot be "sold" to communities; they must be developed by or with real mutual-partnership between the researcher and the communities themselves. Therefore, HIV intervention acceptance in communities begins with the initial development of the interventions. Without community acceptance, translation of effective interventions is likely to be of limited result.

The importance of translating HIV prevention interventions from research settings to routine service delivery has led to the development of an area of research focused on empirically determining the best method for transferring HIV prevention technology (93,94). In the area of HIV transmission risk-reduction research, the science of efficacious interventions has become increasingly refined, particularly in the transfer of interventions to minority and immigrant populations (95). There have been an increasing number of investigations focused on moving the knowledge base from laboratory efficacy studies into real world assessments of these interventions (93,95–98). This action has been supported by the U.S. federal government, which recognizes translational research as a leading priority in the effort to reach these disproportionately affected groups (99). This focus on translational research has been expanded to other realms of research, as illustrated by funding initiatives by various federal institutes (e.g., the Centers for Disease Control and Prevention (CDC), calling for HIV risk-reduction interventions already shown effective for one group to be translated for other groups (100). Translational research must address both language and culture, in terms of substantive adaptations to address the needs and realities of the particular group (101). Specifically, HIV risk-reduction research has focused on how models of change must be expanded and refined to embody the specificities of gender and culture, as well as the physical and social environments facing diverse ethnic groups (102).

Non-governmental organizations are major providers of HIV prevention services, yet their staffs are not necessarily trained in behavior change theories or in how to develop theoretically sound interventions (93,94). Early public health efforts to provide technical assistance weren't comprehensive, tended to be unidirectional, and focused on reducing performance deficits alone, without building performance capacity. As a result of its HIV/AIDS experience, public health agencies like the federal CDC have reconceptualized technical assistance efforts as an endeavor to build capacity. CDC has devised a four-part approach to capacity building: organizational capacity building, intervention technical assistance, community mobilization, and technical assistance in the planning and prioritization of community-based HIV prevention services.

Organizational capacity building refers to strengthening the administrative, human, financial, managerial, and legal resources of the institutions so they are in a position to field effective prevention programs over the short and long term. Intervention technical assistance is the provision of detailed information about the step-by-step implementation of interventions with some empirical basis of effectiveness. Community mobilization (discussed extensively in Chapter 3 of this text) refers to heightening awareness of specific HIV prevention issues and programs within specific communities. And community planning refers to providing the information and skills needed to make informed choices when setting priorities among unmet HIV prevention needs.

Improvements in technical assistance strategies for organizations providing HIV prevention services, brought about by the HIV/AIDS experiences, allow for the building of strong organizations in motivated communities. This particular approach to capacity building could well serve as a model for other public health challenges, beyond the realm of infectious diseases.

Prevention Policy and HIV: Challenges and Solutions

Policy at many levels has affected efforts to prevent HIV transmission. Throughout the epidemic, conflicts about such issues as whether condoms should be distributed in schools, whether sterile injection equipment should be made available for injecting drug users, whether gay bathhouses should be closed down, and whether HIV should be mandatorily reported shaped the way prevention activities have been conducted. Funding to contain the epidemic, both domestically and internationally, has been considered inadequate by many analysts.

However, the HIV epidemic has also produced promising policy shifts, some that may help to reframe our views about health and illness. One notable example, prompted by the epidemic's rapid spread and its increasing toll on human life, is to link our success in dealing with HIV/AIDS to human rights and, more recently, to national security. Such a humanitarian focus of public health is not entirely new. As early as 1946, health was defined by the World Health Organization as "a state of complete physical, mental, and social well-being and not merely an absence of disease or infirmity" (103). Early in the epidemic, various authors and activists pointed to civil and political disparities that increased vulnerability to HIV. Rights to confidentiality, protection from discrimination, access to care—these were all important rallying cries of the gay activist community in the United States in the earliest days of the epidemic. With the rapid spread of this pandemic into poorer communities and developing economies, social and economic inequities were identified as barriers to halting the epidemic. The shift in the epidemic to racial and ethnic minorities (e.g., African Americans accounted for 37 percent of the AIDS cases in the United States in 1999) and women (a tripling in proportion of AIDS cases in the United States from 7 percent in 1985 to 23 percent in 1999) also highlighted the importance of socioeconomic determinates in the United States (14,104). As discussed in Chapters 5 and 7, the HIV/AIDS pandemic has given renewed focus and visibility to the connection between prevention and the promotion of human rights and to the difficulty of the challenge (105–107).

Another very important effect of behavioral intervention research in response to HIV/AIDS has been to highlight the inequities of men and women in most of the world, specifically women's disempowerment in achieving the use of male condoms (108). Concerns that women cannot enforce condom use by their male partners has generated a great deal of energy, activism, and, eventually, research into topical microbicides that might yet become an effective HIV prevention tool that is under women's control (109).

More recently, HIV/AIDS and health more broadly have been tied to national security concerns (see Chapter 9). While the public health danger of STDs was linked to national security interests during both World War I and II, the significance of this threat was minimized with the advent of treatments such as penicillin (110). The lack of an effective HIV-related vaccine, the emergence of new infectious diseases, and microbial resistance to existing antibiotics have all dramatically altered the scenario. The threat from HIV/AIDS has prompted efforts to overcome complacency in the prevention and control of other infectious diseases and to better understand their potential economic, social and political significance both nationally and internationally (111).

Finally, community responses to HIV/AIDS have been instrumental in developing a new era of community involvement and advocacy (see Chapter 3). Activism was not easily accepted or typically a prominent part of traditional "public health practice." But methods developed in response to HIV/AIDS have been highly effective in mobilizing resources, influencing policy, and developing and implementing interventions:

Ultimately, the success of AIDS activist and other advocates for AIDS research funding demonstrated that decisions regarding the allocation of biomedical research resources can be influenced by aggressive and creative lobbying by individuals within and outside the public health community. This lesson has been heeded by advocates for other diseases such as breast cancer, diabetes, and Parkinson disease, and, increasingly by advocates of research for other infectious diseases of global health importance, notably malaria and tuberculosis. (112)

Even bureaucratic, government language regarding public health policy has come to recognize the roles that racism, sexism, and homophobia can play in fueling public health disparities (113).

Many prevention activities now routinely require collaboration and partnership development with organizations not heretofore identified as prevention partners or part of the public health establishment. A CDC HIV prevention initiative, Serostatus Approach to Fighting the Epidemic (SAFE), relies on a public–private partnership of more than fifty organizations, including medical care organizations, the pharmaceutical industry, private industry, the media, and national and community-based HIV prevention organizations (114). And a national plan to eliminate syphilis in the United States, published in late 1999, identifies strengthened community partnerships as an essential national strategy, which is another undeniable legacy of the HIV/AIDS experience (115).

Conclusions

Behavior-change interventions to reduce the risk of HIV transmission have met with unparalleled challenges. There are few infectious agents more insidious than HIV. It is transmitted through the behavior most heavily selected by evolution, sexual intercourse. It is asymptomatic for several years and typically spreads undetected throughout this period. It destroys the body's natural system of defense against disease. It causes many agonizing and terrifying conditions. It is fatal. It targets young adults, the most productive labor resource, resulting in the destruction of national economies of developing countries. Perhaps the only mitigating property of HIV is that it is not casually transmitted.

In this chapter, we have documented some of the positive effects of HIV preventive interventions on intervention research and service provision. We have made significant progress on designing and delivering effective interventions to impoverished, stigmatized, and marginalized populations. We have developed interventions for units greater than the individual, including couples, social groups, and structural interventions that have the capacity to reach entire communities and population groups. In the STD arena, HIV/AIDS has been responsible for a resurgence in health promotion approaches to preventing STD transmission. We have probably developed more prevention capacity in community-based organizations to help deliver HIV interventions than we have for any other public health condition in recent memory. HIV/AIDS has increased the overall behavioral science competence of government—federal, state, and local. We have developed systems of intervention development and prioritization that represent true collaborations between behavioral scientists, health departments, and communities. We look forward to the day that vaccine and other research adds new tools to the armamentarium with which to fight HIV infection.

Acknowledgments

Dr. Malow's contribution was supported in part by RO1 DA09520 from NIDA, R01 AA 013558 from NIAAA, and R01 HD38458 from NICHD. Dr. Holtgrave received support from the Center for AIDS Research at Emory University School of Public Health. The authors wish to thank Ron Valdiserri for many helpful comments and Marie Morgan and Caroline Bailey for editorial assistance.

References

1. Darrow WW, Jaffe HW, and Curran JW: Passive anal intercourse as a risk factor for AIDS in homosexual men. *Lancet* 2(8342): 160, 1983.
2. Centers for Disease Control and Prevention: Immunodeficiency among female sexual partners of males with acquired immune deficiency syndrome (AIDS)—New York [Epidemiologic Notes and Reports]. *Morb Mortal Wkly Rep* 31: 697–698, 1983.
3. Spira TJ, Des Jarlais DC, Marmor M, et al.: Prevalence of antibody to lymphadenopathy-associated virus among drug-detoxification patients in New York [letter]. *N Engl J Med* 311: 467–468, 1984.
4. Valdiserri RO, Lyter DW, Leviton LC, et al.: AIDS prevention in homosexual and bisexual men: results of a randomized trial evaluating two risk reduction interventions. *AIDS* 3: 21–26, 1989.
5. Des Jarlais DC, Casriel C, Friedman SR, and Rosenblum A: AIDS and the transition to illicit drug injection: results of a randomized trial prevention program. *Br J Addiction* 87: 493–498, 1992.
6. National Institutes of Health: Interventions to prevent HIV risk behaviors. *NIH Consensus Statement* 15: 1–41, 1997.
7. Amaro H and Raj A: On the margin: power and women's HIV risk reduction strategies. *Sex Roles* 42(7/8): 723–749, 2000.
8. Canin L, Dolcini M, and Adler N: Barriers to and facilitators of HIV–STD behavior change: intrapersonal and relationship-based factors. *Rev Gen Psychol* 3: 338–371, 1999.
9. Miller M and Neaigus A: Networks, resources and risk among women who use drugs. *Soc Sci Med* 52: 967–978, 2001.
10. O'Leary A and Wingood GM: Interventions for sexually active, heterosexual women. In Peterson JL and DiClemente RJ (ed.): *Handbook of HIV Prevention.* Kluwer/Plenum, New York, 2000, pp. 179–200.
11. Sweat MD and Denison JA: Reducing HIV incidence in developing countries with structural and environmental interventions. *AIDS* 9(suppl A): S251–S257, 1995.
12. Holtgrave DR: Reducing new HIV infections by one-half: what will it take? Putting the goal in historical context, and assessing the cost of unmet needs. Paper presented at the National HIV Prevention Conference, Atlanta, August 12–15, 2001. Abstract 1041.
13. Centers for Disease Control and Prevention: *HIV/AIDS Surveillance Report* 12(2): 1–44, 2001.
14. Centers for Disease Control and Prevention: HIV/AIDS among U.S. women: minority and young women at continuing risk [fact sheet]. Centers for Disease Control and Prevention, Atlanta, September 2000. URL: http://www.cdc.gov/hiv/pubs/facts/women.htm (February 2, 2002).
15. U.S. Department of Health and Human Services: *The Initiative to Eliminate Racial and Ethnic Disparities in Health.* U.S. Department of Health and Human Services, Washington, DC, n.d. URL: http://raceandhealth.hhs.gov (December 15, 2000).
16. Farmer P, Léandreb F, Mukherjeea JS, et al.: Community-based approaches to HIV treatment in resource-poor settings. *Lancet* 358: 404–409, 2001.
17. Sikkema KJ, Kelly JS, Winnett RA, et al.: Outcomes of a randomized community-level HIV prevention intervention for women living in 18 low-income housing developments. *Am J Public Health* 90: 57–63, 2000.

18. St. Lawrence JS, Eldridge GD, Shelby MC, Little CE, Brasfield TL, and O'Bannon RE: HIV risk reduction for incarcerated women: a comparison of brief interventions based on two theoretical models. *J Consult Clin Psychol* 65: 504–509, 1997.

19. Hogben M and St Lawrence JS: Observations from the CDC: HIV/STD risk reduction interventions in prison settings. *J Womens Health Gend Based Med* 9: 587–592, 2000.

20. Fishbein M, Guenther-Grey C, Johnson W, et al.: Using a theory-based community intervention to reduce AIDS risk behaviors: the CDC's AIDS community demonstration projects. In Goldberg ME, Fishbein M, and Middlestat S (eds.): *Social Marketing: Theoretical and Practical Perspectives—Advertising and Consumer Psychology.* Lawrence Erlbaum Associates, Mahwah, NJ, 1997, pp. 123–146.

21. Kamb ML, Fishbein M, Douglas JM Jr, et al.: Efficacy of risk-reduction counseling to prevent human immunodeficiency virus and sexually transmitted diseases: a randomized controlled trial. *JAMA* 280: 1161–1167, 1998.

22. Prendergast ML, Urada D, and Podus D: Meta-analysis of HIV risk-reduction interventions within drug abuse treatment programs. *J Consult Clin Psychol* 69: 389–405, 2001.

23. CDC AIDS Community Demonstration Projects Research Group: Community-level HIV intervention in five cities: final outcome data from the CDC AIDS Community Demonstration Projects. *Am J Public Health* 89: 336–345, 1999.

24. Weissman G and Brown V: Drug-using women and HIV: risk-reduction and prevention issues. In O'Leary A and Jemmott LS (eds.): *Women at Risk: Issues in the Primary Prevention of HIV.* Plenum, New York, 1995, pp. 175–193.

25. Weibel W: *The Indigenous Leader Outreach Model: Intervention Manual* (NIH publication 93-3581). National Institute on Drug Abuse, Rockville, MD, 1993.

26. Kelly JA, Murphy DA, Sikkema KJ, et al.: Randomised, controlled, community-level HIV-prevention intervention for sexual-risk behaviour among homosexual men in US cities: Community HIV Prevention Research Collaborative. *Lancet* 350: 1500–1505, 1997.

27. Greenberg JB and Neumann MS (eds.): *What We Have Learned from the AIDS Evaluation of Street Outreach Projects.* Centers for Disease Control and Prevention, Atlanta, 1998.

28. Resnicow K, Yaroch AL, Davis A, et al.: GO GIRLS! results from a nutrition and physical activity program for low-income, overweight African American adolescent females. *Health Educ Behav* 27: 616–631, 2000.

29. Goldstein KP, Lauderdale DS, Glushak C, Walter J, and Daum RS: Immunization outreach in an inner-city housing development: reminder-recall on foot. *Pediatrics* 104(6): p. 1377, 1999.

30. Miller SK: Nurse practitioners in the county correctional facility setting: unique challenges and suggestions for effective health promotion. *Clinical Excellence for Nurse Practitioners* 3: 268–272, 1999.

31. Roffman RA, Ficciano JF, Ryan R, et al.: HIV-prevention counseling delivered by telephone: an efficacy trial with gay and bisexual men. *AIDS and Behavior* 1: 137–154, 1997.

32. Heckathorn DD: Respondent-driven sampling: a new approach to the study of hidden populations. *Social Problems* 44(2): 174–199, 1997.

33. Latkin CA, Mandell W, Vlahov D, Oziemkowska M, and Celentano DD: The long-term outcome of a personal network-oriented HIV prevention intervention for injection drug users: the SAFE study. *Am J Community Psychol* 24: 341–364, 1996.

34. Rogers EM: Diffusion Theory: A theoretical approach to promote community-level change. Peterson John L and DiClemente Ralph J (eds). (2000) *Handbook of HIV Prevention.* pp. 57–65. New York, NY. Kluwer Academic/Plenum Publishers.

35. O'Leary A, Jemmott LS, Goodhart F, and Gebelt J: Effects of an institutional AIDS prevention intervention: moderation by gender. *AIDS Educ Prev* 8: 49–61, 1996.

36. O'Leary A and Martins P: Structural and policy factors affecting women's HIV risk: a life-course example. *AIDS* 14(suppl): S68–S72, 2000.

37. O'Leary A: Substance use and HIV: disentangling the nexus of risk. *J Subst Abuse* 13: 1–3, 2001.

38. Centers for Disease Control and Prevention: HIV incidence among young men who have sex with men—seven U.S. cities, 1994–2000. *Morb Mortal Wkly Rep* 50: 440–444, 2001.

39. Stall R and Purcell D: Intertwining epidemics: a review of research on substance use among men who have sex with men and its connection to the AIDS epidemic. *AIDS Behav* 4: 181–192, 2000.

40. Hoffman JA, Klein H, Eber M, and Crosby H: Frequency and intensity of crack use as predictors of women's involvement in HIV-related sexual risk behaviors. *Drug Alcohol Depend* 58: 227–236, 2000.

41. Wallace JI, Porter J, Weiner A, and Steinberg A: Oral sex, crack smoking, and HIV infection among female sex workers who do not inject drugs [letter]. *Am J Public Health* 87: 470, 1997.

42. MacDonald TK, MacDonald G, Zanna MP, and Fong G: Alcohol, sexual arousal, and intentions to use condoms in young men: applying alcohol myopia theory to risky sexual behavior. *Health Psychol* 19: 290–298, 2000.

43. Rhodes T, Stimson GV, and Quirk A: Sex, drugs, intervention, and research: from the individual to the social. *Subst Use Misuse* 31: 375–407, 1996.

44. Sloboda Z: What we have learned from research about the prevention of HIV transmission among drug abusers. *Public Health Rep* 113(suppl 1): 194–204, 1998.

45. Kalichman SC, Hunter TL, and Kelley JA: Perceptions of AIDS susceptibility among minority and nonminority women at risk for HIV infection. *J Consult Clin Psychol* 60: 725–732, 1992.

46. Barthwell A: African American women and drug-related HIV infection and AIDS. Center for Substance Abuse Prevention. *Prev Monogr* 13: 113–129, 1993.

47. Kalichman SC, Adair V, Somlai AM, and Weir SS: The perceived social context of AIDS: study of inner-city sexually transmitted disease clinic patients. *AIDS Educ Prev* 7: 298–307, 1995

48. Wingood GM and DiClemente RJ: Consequences of having a physically abusive partner on condom use and sexual negotiation of young adult African-American women. *Am J Public Health* 87: 1016–1018, 1997.

49. Kalichman SC, Williams EA, Cherry C, Belcher L, and Nachimson D: Sexual coercion, domestic violence, and negotiating condom use among low-income African American women. *J Women's Health* 7: 371–378, 1998.

50. Ickovics JR, Hamburger ME, Vlahov D, et al.: Mortality, CD4 decline, and depressive symptoms among HIV-seropositive women: longitudinal analysis from the HIV Epidemiology Research Study. *JAMA* 285: 1466–1474, 2001.

51. Malow RM, Corigan S, Pena J, Calkins A, and Bannister T: Mood and HIV risk behavior among drug dependent veterans. *Psychol Addict Behav* 2: 131–134, 1992.

52. Lucenko BA, Malow RM, Sanchez-Martinez M, Jennings T, Dévieux JG, and Kalich-

man S: Negative affect and HIV risk in alcohol and other drug (AOD) abusing adolescent offenders. *J Child Adolesc Subst Abuse.* In press.

53. Bonin MF, McCreary DR, and Sadava SW: Problem drinking behavior in two community-based samples of adults: influence of gender, coping, loneliness, and depression. *Psychol Addict Behav* 14(2): 151–161, 2000.

54. Newacheck PW, Halfon N, Brindis CD, and Hughes DC: Evaluating community efforts to decategorize and integrate financing of children's health services. *Milbank Q* 76(2): 157–173, 1998.

55. Schneir A, Kipke MD, Melchior LA, and Huba GJ: Children's Hospital Los Angeles: a model of integrated care for HIV-positive and very high-risk youth. *J Adolesc Health* 23(2 suppl): 59–70, 1998.

56. Grossman JB and Sipe CL: *Summer Training and Education Program (STEP): Report on Long-term Impacts.* Public/Private Ventures, Philadelphia, 1992.

57. O'Donnell L, Stueve A, Dovan AS, et al.: The effectiveness of the Reach for Health community youth service learning program in reducing early and unprotected sex among urban middle-school students. *Am J Public Health* 89: 176–181, 1999.

58. Purcell DW, DeGroff A, and Wolitski RJ: HIV prevention case management: current practice and future directions. *Health Soc Work* 23: 282–289, 1998.

59. Katz MH, Cunningham WE, Fleishman JA, et al.: Effect of case management on unmet needs and utilization of medical care and medications among HIV-infected persons [see comments]. *Ann Intern Med* 135(8 pt 1): 557–565, 2001.

60. Diefenbach MA and Leventhal H: The common-sense model of illness representation: theoretical and practical considerations. *J Soc Distress Homeless* 5(1): 11–38, 1996.

61. Gold RS, Skinner MJ, and Ross MW: Unprotected anal intercourse in HIV-infected and non-HIV-infected gay men. *J Sex Res* 31: 59–77, 1994.

62. Suarez T and Miller J: Negotiating risks in context: a perspective on unprotected anal intercourse and barebacking among men who have sex with men—where do we go from here? *Arch Sex Behav* 30(3): 655–669, 2001.

63. Wolitski RJ and Branson BM: Grey area behaviors and partner selection strategies. In O'Leary A (ed.): *Beyond Condoms: Alternative Approaches to HIV Prevention.* Kluwer Academic/Plenum, New York, 2002, pp. 173–199.

64. Kippax S: Negotiated safety agreements among gay men. In O'Leary A (ed.): *Beyond Condoms: Alternative Approaches to HIV Prevention.* Kluwer Academic/Plenum, New York, 2002, pp. 1–15.

65. O'Leary A (ed.): *Beyond Condoms: Alternative Approaches to HIV Prevention.* Kluwer Academic/Plenum, New York, 2002.

66. Hanenberg RS, Rojanapithayakorn W, Kunasol P, et al.: Impact of Thailand's HIV control program as indicated by the decline of sexually transmitted diseases. *Lancet* 344: 243–245, 1994.

67. Albert AE, Warner DL, Hatcher RA, Trussell J, and Bennett C: Condom use among female commercial sex workers in Nevada's legal brothels. *Am J Public Health* 85: 1514–1520, 1995.

68. Aral SO and Peterman TA: STD diagnosis and treatment as an HIV prevention strategy. In O'Leary A (ed.): *Beyond Condoms: Alternative Approaches to HIV Prevention.* Kluwer Academic/Plenum, New York, 2002, pp. 77–90.

69. Des Jarlais DC, Guydish J, Friedman SR, and Hagan H: HIV/AIDS prevention for drug users in natural settings. In Peterson JL and DiClemente RJ (eds.): *Handbook of HIV Prevention.* Kluwer Academic/Plenum, New York, 2000, pp. 159–177.

70. Morin SF: Early detection of HIV: assessing the legislative context. *J Acquire Immune Defic Syndr* 25(suppl 2): S144–S150, 2000.

71. Chesson HW, Harrison P, and Kassler WJ: Sex under the influence: the effect of alcohol policy on sexually transmitted disease rates in the United States. *J Law Econ* 43: 215–238, 2000.

72. Centers for Disease Control and Prevention: Alcohol policy and sexually transmitted disease rates—United States, 1981–1995. *Morb Mortal Wkly Rep* 49: 346–349, 2000.

73. Fried CS: Juvenile curfews: are they an effective and constitutional means of combating juvenile violence? *Behav Sci Law* 19(1): 127–141, 2001.

74. Battle EK and Brownell KD: Confronting a rising tide of eating disorders and obesity: treatment vs prevention and policy. *Addict Behav* 21: 755–765, 1996.

75. Horgen KB and Brownell KD: Policy change as a means for reducing the prevalence and impact of alcoholism, smoking, and obesity. In Miller WR and Heather N (eds.): *Treating Addictive Behaviors,* 2nd ed. (Applied Clinical Psychology Series). Plenum, New York, 1998, pp. 105–118.

76. Roberts LJ and Marlatt GA: Harm reduction. In Ott PJ, Tarter RE, Tarter R, and Ammerman R (eds.): *Sourcebook on Substance Abuse: Etiology, Epidemiology, Assessment, and Treatment.* Allyn and Bacon, Needham Heights, Mass., 1999, pp. 389–398.

77. Hamilton M: Researching harm-reduction care and contradictions. *Subst Use Misuse* 34: 119–141, 1999.

78. Larimer ME, Marlatt GA, Baer JS, Quigley LA, Blume AW, and Hawkins EH. Harm reduction for alcohol problems: expanding access to and acceptability of prevention and treatment services. In Marlatt GA (ed.): *Harm Reduction: Pragmatic Strategies for Managing High-Risk Behaviors.* Guilford, New York, 1998, pp. 69–121.

79. Baer JS and Murch HB: Harm reduction, nicotine, and smoking. In Marlatt GA (ed.): *Harm Reduction: Pragmatic Strategies for Managing High-Risk Behaviors.* Guilford, New York, 1998, pp. 122–144.

80. Fisher JD and Fisher WA: Theoretical approaches to individual-level change in HIV risk behavior. In Peterson JL and DiClemente, RJ (eds.): *Handbook of HIV Prevention.* Kluwer Academic/Plenum, New York, 2000, pp. 3–55.

81. Peterson JL and DiClemente RJ (eds.): *Handbook of HIV Prevention.* Kluwer Academic/Plenum, New York, 2000.

82. Roth DL, Stewart KE, Clay OJ, van der Straten A, Karita E, and Allen S: Sexual practices of HIV discordant and concordant couples in Rwanda: effects of a testing and counseling programme for men. *Int J STD AIDS* 12: 181–188, 2001.

83. The Voluntary HIV-1 Counseling and Testing Efficacy Study Group: Efficacy of Voluntary HIV-1 Counselling and Testing in Individuals and Couples in Kenya, Tanzania and Trinidad: A randomised trial. *Lancet* 358: 103–112, 2000.

84. Carballo-Dieguez A and Remien RH: Sex therapy with male couples of mixed-(serodiscordant-) HIV status. In Kleinplatz PJ (ed.): *New Directions in Sex Therapy: Innovations and Alternatives.* Brunner-Routledge, Philadelphia, 2001, pp. 302–321.

85. Buchacz K, van der Straten A, Saul J, Shiboski S, Gomez C, and Padian N: Behavioral, sociodemographic, and clinical correlates of inconsistent condom use in HIV-serodiscordant heterosexual couples. *J Acquir Immune Defic Syndr* 28: 289–297, 2001.

86. El-Bassel N: Couple-based HIV/STD prevention for heterosexual couples recruited from a primary health-care setting. In Pequegnat W (chair): *Symposium on Design-*

ing More Effective AIDS Prevention Programs for Women and Families; 2001 National HIV Prevention Conference; August 12–15, 2001, Atlanta. Abstract 922.

87. Miller KS, Levin ML, Whitaker DJ, and Xu X. Patterns of condom use among adolescents: the impact of mother–adolescent communication. *Am J Public Health* 88: 1542–1544, 1998.

88. Rankin-Esquer L, Deeter AK, Froelicher E, and Taylor C: Coronary heart disease: intervention for intimate relationship issues. *Cognit Behav Pract* 7: 212–220, 2000.

89. Taylor CB, Bandura A, Ewart CK, Miller NH, and DeBusk RF: Exercise testing to enhance wives' confidence in their husbands' capability soon after clinically uncomplicated myocardial infarction. *Am J Cardiol* 55: 635–638, 1985.

90. Fals-Stewart W, Birchler GR, and O'Farrell TJ: Behavioral couples therapy for male substance-abusing patients: effects on relationship adjustment and drug-using behavior. *J Consult Clin Psychol* 64: 959–972, 1996.

91. Kang SH, Bloom JR, and Romano PS: Cancer screening among African-American women: their use of tests and social support. *Am J Public Health* 84: 101–103.

92. Lamb S, Greenlick MR, and McCarty D: (Committee on Community-Based Drug Treatment, Institute of Medicine) (eds.): *Bridging the Gap between Practice and Research: Forging Partnerships with Community-Based Drug and Alcohol Treatment.* National Academy Press, Washington, DC, 1998.

93. Kelly JA, Somlai AM, DiFrancesico WJ, et al.: Bridging the gap between the science and service of HIV prevention: transferring effective research-based HIV prevention interventions to community AIDS service providers. *Am J Public Health* 90: 1082–1088, 2000.

94. DiFrancesico W, Kelly JA, Otto-Salaj L, et al.: Factors influencing attitudes within AIDS service organizations toward the use of research-based HIV prevention interventions. *AIDS Educ Prev* 11(1): 72–86, 1999.

95. Malow R, Rosenberg R, and Devieux J: Translating primary HIV prevention intervention in diverse groups: the AIDS Prevention Center (APC) in Miami. *Psychol AIDS Exchange* 28: 1–8, 2000.

96. Kelly JA, Sogolow ED, and Neumann MS: Future directions and emerging issues in technology transfer between HIV prevention researchers and community-based service providers. *AIDS Educ Prev* 12: 126–141, 2000.

97. Rotheram-Borus MJ: Expanding the range of interventions to reduce HIV among adolescents. *AIDS* 14(suppl 1): 33–40, 2000.

98. Malow R, Dévieux JG, Rosenberg R, Capp L, and Schneiderman N: A cognitive-behavioral intervention for HIV+ recovering drug abusers: the 2000–05 NIDA-funded AIDS Prevention Center study. *Psychol AIDS Exchange* 30: 23–26, 2001.

99. National Institutes of Health, Office of AIDS Research: *Minority Initiatives,* n.d. URL: http://www.nih.gov/od/oar/minority/minority.htm (February 26, 2002).

100. Neumann MS and Sogolow ED: Replicating effective programs: HIV/AIDS prevention technology transfer. *AIDS Educ Prev* 12(suppl A): 35–48, 2000.

101. Resnicow K, Baranowski T, Ahluwalia JS, and Braithwaite RL: Cultural sensitivity in public health: defined and demystified. *Ethn Dis* 9(1): 10–21, 1999.

102. Ortiz-Torres B, Serrano-Garcia I, and Torres-Burgos N: Subverting culture: promoting HIV/AIDS prevention among Puerto Rican and Dominican women. *Am J Community Psychol* 28: 859–881, 2000.

103. World Health Organization: *Official Record,* Vol 2. World Health Organization, Geneva, 1946, p. 100.

104. Centers for Disease Control and Prevention: *HIV/AIDS among African Americans*

[fact sheet]. Centers for Disease Control and Prevention, Atlanta, September 2000. URL: http://www.cdc.gov/hiv/pubs/facts/afam.htm (Feburary 2, 2002).

105. Heywood M and Altman D: Confronting AIDS: human rights, law and social transformation. *Health Hum Rights* 5(1): 149–179, 2000.

106. Mann JM: Medicine and public health, ethics and human rights. *Hastings Cent Rep* 27(3): 6–13, 1997.

107. Mann JM: Health and human rights [editorial]. *Br Med J* 312: 924–925, 1996.

108. Gupta GR and Weiss E: Women's lives and sex: implications for AIDS prevention. *Cult Med Psychiatry* 17: 399–412, 1993.

109. Moore JS and Rogers M: Female-controlled prevention technologies. In O'Leary A (ed.): *Beyond Condoms: Alternative Approaches to HIV Prevention.* Kluwer Academic/Plenum, New York, 2002, pp. 47–76.

110. Vermund SH and Fawal H. Emerging infectious diseases and professional integrity: thoughts for the new millennium. *Am J Infect Control* 27: 497–499, 1999.

111. Piot P, Bartos M, Ghys PD, Walker N, and Schwartzlander B: The global impact of HIV/AIDS. *Nature* 410: 968–973, 2001.

112. Folkers GK and Fauci AS: The AIDS research model: implications for other infectious diseases of global health importance. *JAMA* 286: 458–461, 2001.

113. Mitka M: U.S. effort to eliminate syphilis moving forward. *JAMA* 283: 1555–1556, 2000.

114. Janssen RS, Holtgrave DR, Valdiserri RO, Shepherd M, Gayle HD, and De Cock KM: The serostatus approach to fighting the HIV epidemic: prevention strategies for infected individuals. *Am J Public Health* 91: 1019–1024, 2001.

115. Centers for Disease Control and Prevention: *The National Plan to Eliminate Syphilis from the United States.* Centers for Disease Control and Prevention, Atlanta, 1999. URL: http://www.cdc.gov/stopsyphilis (December 1, 2000).

5

The Impact of HIV/AIDS on the Development of Public Health Law

SCOTT BURRIS AND LAWRENCE O. GOSTIN

Public health law is the study of the legal powers and duties of the state to assure the conditions for people to be healthy (e.g., to identify, prevent, and ameliorate risks to the health of the populations) and the limitations on the power of the state to constrain the autonomy, privacy, liberty, proprietary, or other legally protected interests of individuals for the protection or promotion of community health.

(1: 4)

When the United States was struck by a serious epidemic of HIV/AIDS in the early 1980s, public health law was an all but abandoned field. For decades, communicable disease had been in decline, and with it the use of various powers the law had long ago given to health agencies charged with controlling those diseases. In a world in which chronic noncommunicable diseases, accidents, and environmental toxins dominated the health concerns of the U.S. public and policymakers, and in which the few residual communicable diseases were susceptible to treatment and largely untroubling to society, there was little occasion for the use or renewal of a body of law whose time was thought to be past—if, indeed, it was thought about at all.

Lawyers responding to the public health issues raised by the AIDS epidemic found many symptoms of this long disuse. Faced with proposals to "quarantine" people with HIV, lawyers had to go back to 1905 to find the "leading" Supreme Court case on coercive public health measures, a case that dealt with compulsory smallpox vaccination in the face of an actual epidemic (2). Early commentators in HIV law typically found themselves relying far more heavily on nineteenth- and early-twentieth-century cases about smallpox, cholera, tuberculosis, and yellow fever than any contemporary decisions (3,4). The public health law treatises then in print were more focused on health care or the important, but rather routine, administrative aspects of public health powers as applied to matters like restaurant inspection (5,6,7). For detailed technical discussion of public health law issues, lawyers found themselves among the antiquities of the law library, drawing on James Tobey's work of the 1930s (8), and even nineteenth-century texts like Parker and Worthington on public health law (9), *Cooley on Constitutional Limitations* (10), and Ernst Freund's (11) and Christopher Tiedeman's (12) works on the police power.

Statutes setting out the powers of health agencies were equally venerable. Lawyers were surprised to find basic public health statutes that had not been revised for decades, which gave health departments powers they no longer used, and allowed them to infringe the liberties of individuals under procedures that failed to reflect the substantial developments of constitutional law in the decades following World War II (3,13). Validating this impression, the Institute of Medicine's (IOM) 1988 report on *The Future of Public Health* concluded that "this nation has lost sight of its public health goals and has allowed the system of public health activities to fall into disarray." The IOM placed some of the blame on an obsolete and inadequate body of enabling laws and regulations (14) and recommended that

states review their public health statutes and make revisions necessary to accomplish the following two objectives: [i] clearly delineate the basic authority and responsibility entrusted to public health agencies, boards, and officials at the state and local levels and the relationship between them; and [ii] support a set of modern disease control measures that address contemporary health problems such as AIDS, cancer, and heart disease, and incorporate due process safeguards (notice, hearings, administrative review, right to counsel, standards of evidence). (14: 10)

Historically, public health law has been shaped by the social response to serious epidemics. Boards of health and full-fledged health departments were created in the late eighteenth and early nineteenth centuries in response to yellow fever and cholera (15,16,17). Disease reporting, mandatory screening, and compulsory treatment became common in the law in response to tuberculosis (18) and syphilis (19). HIV proved to be no exception. The need to respond, and the special role of law as a medium for resolving social disputes in the United States, gave public health law a renewed importance. Advocates turned to law as a tool for promoting their desired HIV policies. Lawyers, judges, policy-makers, and public health officials were challenged to adapt old practices to new needs and to develop new solutions to new problems. In the process, public health law has reemerged as a vital discipline of public health, with a stronger connection to practice and a deeper intellectual foundation.

After a brief overview of the statutes and cases arising from the epidemic, this chapter describes how HIV/AIDS perfected a change in the use of public health power. In the face of HIV/AIDS, public health has accepted the limits of law as a means to coerce behavior change among people with or at risk of communicable disease; at the same time, it has become more interested in understanding and addressing how law contributes to the social conditions in which people would be most likely to behave in healthy ways. The chapter focuses on two examples of this change in practice: the effort to use law to reduce social risk, and the development and application of a human rights framework in public health practice. The chapter concludes with some thoughts on the influence of HIV/AIDS on the future course of law in public health.

Overview of Case Law

The first case directly involving HIV to go to trial, in 1983, was an unsuccessful effort by New York state prison inmates to force the state to segregate prisoners with HIV (20). Official public health efforts to control HIV first took legal form in late 1984, when San Francisco Health Commissioner Mervyn Silverman went to court for an order closing down bathhouses and other businesses where, he alleged, unsafe sexual activity was posing a serious threat of HIV transmission (4). At about the same time, a few school districts across the country refused admission to children with HIV on health grounds, leading to a series of important cases under federal and state antidiscrimination law establishing that HIV is a protected disability (21,22,23). During the late 1980s and early 1990s, the growing social encounter with HIV produced a wide range of disputes over matters that included the rights of prisoners with HIV (24); civil liability for negligently transmitting or exposing others to HIV through sex, blood transfusion, or health-care activities (25); criminal responsibility for transmitting or attempting to transmit HIV (26); parenting rights of people with HIV (27); breach of privacy (28); discrimination in employment (22), insurance (29), health care (30), and housing (31); and improper or involuntary HIV testing (28,32). In one case of particular public health interest, a group of New York physicians unsuccessfully asked a court to force the state health commissioner to categorize HIV as a sexually transmitted disease, which would have triggered various measures (such as name reporting) that the commissioner considered inadvisable (33). HIV/AIDS discrimination and privacy cases remained important parts of the litigation picture as the 1990s went on, but there was a significant infusion of personal injury litigation based on exposure or fear of exposure to the virus in health-care settings (34–37). By 1998, there had been over 1,000 lawsuits raising significant issues related to HIV (38,39), enough activity to support AIDS legal assistance organizations in most major U.S. cities, a legal periodical devoted solely to AIDS litigation (40), and a regularly updated legal treatise (41).

These early cases reaffirmed some enduring baselines in U.S. legal doctrine and set some new ones. Broadly speaking, people with HIV are entitled to protection of their privacy and to be free from discrimination in employment, housing, and access to services. People who deliberately or recklessly endangered others through HIV exposure are subject to prosecution under traditional criminal laws and could be liable for civil damages in tort. Suppliers of blood and blood products have generally not been liable for transfusion-associated HIV under either negligence or product liability theories. Federal agencies do not violate the Constitution by screening employees or participants in programs, like the Job Corps, for HIV, despite the general illegality of such screening in the private sector. Most important for public health agencies, the cases generally upheld the authority of health officials to take action to protect the public against significant risks of HIV transmission, even when action infringed on constitutionally protected rights, and required courts to defer to the reasoned judgments of health officials (42).

The court system is a forum for airing and sometimes resolving important individual and social disputes arising from HIV/AIDS. Litigation is an imperfect mirror in which to view either social policy or social phenomena, however. Judicial decisions often get considerable attention, but the type and distribution of disputes in court generally bears no direct relationship to disputes and behavior in the world. It is well known that only a small proportion of people who have disputes that could be resolved through legal action take these disputes to court (43,44) and, at the other end of the process, that one cannot safely generalize from the nonrandom and very small subset of cases that produce a published opinion or well-publicized trial (45). For example, in the case of HIV/AIDS, reviewing court records does not provide an accurate measure of how frequently people with HIV suffer discrimination or breach of privacy (30).

Overview of Legislation and Regulation

The drama of litigation should not divert attention from the legislative and administrative processes that are the true engines of law as a tool of public health policy. As we will discuss, HIV occasioned a dramatic, even unprecedented, level of advocacy and legislative debate about the full range of policies related to HIV, including topics as diverse as the basic powers of health departments, the regulation of insurance, the approval of new drugs, the prevention of discrimination, the content of HIV education, medical privacy, and the operation of the social security disability system. The outcomes have been equally diverse. Legislatures have generally protected the social status of people with and at risk of the disease, but they have also passed laws criminalizing various kinds of HIV-related behavior. HIV advocates have created a model for disease-based lobbying, securing a high level of funding for research and care, but have frequently lost battles on issues like HIV reporting and needle exchange, and they face even greater competition for scarce dollars in the aftermath of the September 11, 2001, attacks on the United States (46).

The first great wave of HIV legislation in the states established basic rules of informed consent for HIV testing and the confidentiality of HIV test results and other medical information (28). By the end of the 1980s, most states had laws of this kind in place (47,48). State legislatures generally left the decisions about what basic control measure to implement to health agencies, which then implemented name-based reporting of AIDS, partner notification, and personal control measures under existing statutory authority, with little or no interference from courts (49,50). In some instances, however, legislatures required HIV reporting, banned anonymous testing, or passed statutes that set new procedures for dealing with HIV risk behavior (51). Illinois's legislature mandated premarital screening, which was repealed after a year's experience showed it to be a costly failure (52). Utah's legislature went so far as to ban marriage between HIV positive people altogether, a statute that was quickly declared unconstitutional (53). In recent years, the question of whether to liberalize syringe access to prevent HIV has been taken up by legislatures across the country, with a variety of results (54).

Many states, by statute or administrative action, required the provision of HIV education in schools. Several states require education about HIV and testing to be distributed to marriage license applicants or to individuals charged with prostitution or drug-related crimes (48). A 1990 Philadelphia ordinance, of more symbolic than practical effect, required any employer of three or more people to provide oral HIV education, by a senior management official, to employees (55).

The federal government, whose role in public health law is constitutionally secondary to that of the states (1), tended to have its influence through a combination of primarily voluntary standard setting, through the Centers for Disease Control and Prevention (CDC), and in the exercise of its spending power. CDC guidelines on all manner of issues, from educating kids with HIV at schools to how to deal with HIV-infected health-care workers, were frequently cited by judges and deferred to by legislators (56). Through its power to place conditions on funding, Congress periodically accomplished considerable control over various aspects of HIV policy. Notably, Senator Jesse Helms sponsored a series of amendments to appropriations bills, limiting the content of federally funded HIV education materials. Although some of these restrictions were invalidated by courts (55), CDC funding is still subject to congressional content guidelines.

Appropriations riders were also used to nudge states into passing criminal provisions. For example, in 1990, Congress enacted federal legislation that required states to provide mandatory testing programs for convicted sex offenders in order to qualify for federal funds (57). An ongoing ban on the use of federal funds to support needle exchange programs for injecting drug users not only was an important political symbol in the battle over the legalization of such programs but also may have deterred public health agencies and community-based organizations from providing syringe access services even where they were legal. At the administrative level, ACT-UP spearheaded a successful effort to speed the approval of new drugs by the FDA, and increase access to investigational drugs (58), while benefits advocates were able to persuade the Social Security Administration to make an AIDS diagnosis presumptive evidence of disability and, after a long battle, broaden the agency's approach to defining AIDS (59).

The federal government's own legal actions sometimes constituted significant public health measures. Perhaps the most notable example was the bloodborne pathogen standard issued by OSHA in 1991, which mandated the use of universal infection-control precautions where there was a risk of occupational exposure to blood (60). Moreover, the federal government has both extensive management responsibilities over its own operations and public health responsibilities connected with immigration and foreign relations. The U.S. government moved early in the epidemic to screen and exclude HIV-positive military recruits, Job Corps applicants, new State Department employees, and immigrants (32).

Reassessing the Role of Law in Public Health: From Coercion to Structural Interventions

As this brief overview has suggested, HIV has brought both a reaffirmation of the legal authority of health officials to take coercive measures in the course of disease control and a much clearer recognition of the limits of coercion, both legal and practical. Indeed, the focus of public health law has moved to a considerable degree during the epidemic from law as simply a tool for forcing certain recalcitrant people to change their behavior, to law as a structural factor that contributes to population vulnerability and as a mode of structural intervention to help create the conditions in which people can make healthier choices (61).

Coercion—behavioral commands backed by the power of the state—is an important tool of public health and has been deployed in HIV control. Individuals deemed to pose risks of transmission to others have been presented with court or administrative orders to modify their behavior; some have been confined. Half the states have passed laws explicitly authorizing coercive measures against people with HIV who endangered others (48,62), and the general power to take such action is part of every state's law (13). People who exposed others to HIV have been convicted of crimes and imprisoned (63). As described in this chapter, people in some states have been required to undergo HIV testing as a condition of getting a marriage license, entering certain government programs and agencies, and upon arrest or conviction of certain crimes. People have also been legally denied certain kinds of employment because of the supposed risk of transmission (64). Less coercively, but still intrusively, states have required information about a person's disease status to be reported to the health department, and they have routinely asked individuals newly diagnosed with HIV to identify their partners for notification. In nearly all instances, the exercise of this power was upheld by courts—or simply not challenged (3).

Although it is legal, the exercise of coercive powers by health agencies against people with HIV has been infrequent. Bayer and Fairchild-Carino's study of health department activities between 1981 and 1990 found only ten instances of HIV-related quarantine. Twenty-four state health departments either had no mechanism for taking reports from the public of unsafe individual behavior or took no action upon such reports (62). Gellert and colleagues, describing the experiences of Orange County's program for addressing reports of unsafe HIV-related behavior, reported that all the HIV-positive people it had found necessary to confine were experiencing acute mental illness and were committed for treatment under the mental health, rather than public health, law (65). Health authorities in several major cities took action against public sex venues. San Francisco's early attempt at outright closure of sex venues gave way to a system of self-regulation. In New York, ongoing health department monitoring led to periodic closure actions (66).

Notwithstanding the occasional exercise of coercive powers by health authorities, the HIV epidemic saw the development of a voluntarist consensus whose central tenet was that HIV control could not succeed without the voluntary cooperation of those with and at risk of infection. The consensus was incomplete but influential, manifested legally in the widespread support of public health authorities for confidentiality laws, limits on HIV testing, protection against discrimination, caution in the introduction of named HIV reporting, and disinclination to use measures like isolation or to turn matters over to the criminal justice system (67,68). This consensus was supported by the reports of expert panels (69) and national commissions on HIV (70). Internationally, the consensus is seen most clearly in the work of the U.N. AIDS programs fostering a "human rights" approach to global HIV control (71).

The voluntarist rationale reached its legal apogee in the case of *School Board of Nassau County v. Arline*, in which the U.S. Supreme Court ruled that the nation's disability discrimination law protected people with communicable diseases from unjustified discrimination, even if it came at the behest of a public health official (72,73). Gene Arline, a teacher with tuberculosis, was dismissed by her school board, on the recommendation of the local TB control officer. The *Arline* Court took it as a given that people with communicable disease have no "right" to endanger others and that the state has the obligation to prevent disease. The job of the law is to "protect handicapped individuals from deprivations based on prejudice, stereotypes, or unfounded fear, while giving appropriate weight to such legitimate concerns . . . as avoiding exposing others to significant health and safety risks" (72: 287). Challenges to discriminatory actions, including public health measures, thus impose on courts the task of determining when discrimination is justified. The court provided the answer: such treatment could only be justified if Ms. Arline was shown by competent medical evidence to pose a significant risk—that is, a "high probability of substantial harm" (74)—to others in the school. The determination that a person poses a direct threat to the health or safety of others may not be based on generalizations or stereotypes about a particular disability. Rather, the determination must be based on an individualized assessment of the risk that the person poses and on reasonable judgments that reflect current scientific data or other objective evidence: "In making these findings, courts should normally defer to the reasonable medical judgments of public health officials" (72: 288).

William Rehnquist, in dissent, protested that this decision would interfere with the ability of state and local health officials to protect the public from communicable disease. Justice Brennan's reply, for the majority of the Court, captured the essence of the voluntarist approach:

Conforming employment decisions with medically reasonable judgments can hardly be thought to threaten the States' regulation of communicable diseases. Indeed, because the Act requires employers to respond rationally to those handicapped by a contagious disease, the Act will assist local health officials by helping remove an important obstacle to preventing the spread of infectious diseases: the individual's reluctance to report his or her condition. (72: 286–287 n. 15)

A few states amended their basic public health statutes to give health authorities an explicit set of increasingly coercive options for dealing with individuals who were posing health threats, consistent with this voluntarist consensus. These statutes were premised on the basic principle of "least restrictive means," under which the least coercive and intrusive measure that would be effective was always required to be chosen. These statutes also tended to adopt Arline's "significant risk" requirement as the threshold for action. In the majority of states, this general approach was adopted without explicit changes in health statutes. Our 1998 review of statutes found that while HIV changed how public health officials exercised their coercive powers, and helped clarify the effect of new law on old practices, the statutory base of public health remained outmoded (13).

Voluntarism, and particularly caution in the deployment of coercion, had many roots. One, certainly, was political engagement by gay people, who united in effective advocacy organizations that supported the passage of protective legislation, demanded funding for research and treatment, and opposed coercive and punitive measures (68,75). The role of law in limiting resort to coercion in HIV/AIDS control should also not be underestimated. The *Arline* case was important in confirming the applicability of disability law to coercive public health measures aimed at communicable disease. But its core approach—requiring that actions taken against people with communicable disabilities be based on a demonstrated significant risk—was consistent with the general need-based approach of courts in the older public health cases (4,76,77). Conservatism in the application of coercion certainly also reflected the greater protection afforded individual rights in post–World War II jurisprudence (3).

Public health officials, mindful of the legal importance of individual rights, were likely hesitant to tangle with a well-organized and vociferous group of advocates. More important, however, public health professionals had independently come to rely very little on coercive measures. Despite the claim of some people that HIV was being treated "differently" because of the avoidance of isolation and mandatory testing, the use of coercion had been in decline for two or three decades across the range of communicable diseases (19,78,79) From a public health point of view, this decline reflected good sense and practical experience rather than political accommodation.

Indeed, the emerging HIV epidemic was ill-suited to a coercive response for at least two important practical reasons. One might be called the "not-enough-policemen" problem. With hundreds of thousands of people already infected by the mid-1980s, and these infections occurring through private, voluntary behaviors that are highly gratifying, it was very unlikely that society could "arrest" its way out of the epidemic. Deterrence had done very little to reduce homosexuality, prostitution, or drug use. Were HIV being spread by a small number of readily identifiable people, coercive action against those individuals might have been indicated and justifiable by necessity; low prevalence and treatability were among the reasons that directly observed therapy and even long-term confinement were instituted in TB control (80,81). Changing the private behaviors of millions of people in populations at risk is a much taller order, and one in which the direct exercise of coercive power on each individual is impractical if not repugnant.

The second reason followed from the first. If safe behavior could not be coerced, it had to be encouraged, even facilitated. Early in the epidemic, when the prevention emphasis was almost entirely on individually oriented educational and motivational interventions, health authorities needed the help and support of communities at risk in order to craft and effectively deliver acceptable messages; this imperative increased in the mid-1980s when antibody testing came into use. Gaining this support—at both the individual and community level—certainly entailed avoiding unnecessary exercise of coercive authority, along with a general support for voluntarist responses. As experience grew, it became increasingly clear that individual behavior change depended to a considerable degree on the cues and options individuals face at the partner, community, and societal level and that law was an important tool for influencing the social environment (82).

At the community and population levels, law's importance as a tool of individual coercion is far less significant a factor in public health than its role in structuring current behavioral options and its potential use as an intervention to change community and social level norms and practices (61,82). Commentators have described significant instances, such as the campaign against smoking, in which law was used to change behavior less by specific regulation than by changing its "social meaning" (83,84). In the HIV epidemic, law in its structuring role has both increased vulnerability—for example, by limiting drug users' access to sterile injection equipment (85)—and been deployed to support voluntary behavioral change efforts: for example, by protecting people who get tested from discrimination (86).

As we emerge from the second decade of the epidemic in the United States, coercion remains a necessary weapon in the public health arsenal. But as this discussion has shown, its use as the default mode of public health response is not necessarily positive. Of much greater salience is the role of law in inadvertently facilitating unhealthy behaviors and outcomes, as well as the use of law as a tool of positive intervention in promoting healthy behaviors. The next two sections of this chapter look more closely at the two major efforts to use law to provide social conditions supportive of HIV prevention: the legal campaign to protect people with HIV from social risks, and the health and human rights movement. We ask how they have influenced public health so far and what they bode for future public health practice.

Addressing Social Risk as a Public Health Problem: Work in Progress

The commitment to voluntarism entailed both conservatism in the use of individual coercion and an effort to deal with the social factors that could deter people from being tested for HIV or otherwise cooperating with public health efforts (75,86). From early in the epidemic, concerns about discrimination, prejudice, and stigma were taken quite seriously by public health officials and policy-makers. In the law, these concerns were reflected in the unprecedented level of privacy and antidiscrimination protection for people with HIV, as well as in the attention paid over the years to mitigating the effects of employment problems on insurance access (29) and portability (87). The urgency of addressing social risks was also seen to shape the international response to HIV (25,88) and became essentially an "article of faith" in the emerging discussion of the public health response to advances in genetics (89,90). In hindsight, the effort to address social risk can be seen as an ambitious structural intervention using law to create social conditions in which voluntarist HIV prevention efforts were most likely to succeed.

Concern with social matters generally and the influence of social attitudes on the behavior of people with diseases is not new in public health (19,78,79), but as a result of the HIV experience, dealing with social risk is now clearly a more prominent part of the basic public health agenda. It is important not to underestimate the extent to which the legal response to HIV—in both legislation and litigation—has been driven by the imperative to protect people against at least some social risks. One might say that the *Arline* case represents the official acceptance of a rational, humane response to communicable disease that truly did turn its back on centuries of reflexive disease isolationism. Yet precisely because the widespread acceptance of nondiscrimination and other positive responses to social risk is an important result of HIV, we need to assess it.

That bad social consequences are more or less likely to flow from being identified as HIV positive is another of the abiding truisms of the epidemic. In fact, however, the nature and extent of the problem remain, after two decades, drastically underresearched and even undefined. There are few data on the incidence of discrimination or breach of privacy related to HIV serostatus (30,91). More important, it is not clear why, apart from their fit with legal available "solutions," we should conceive of the social vulnerability occasioned by HIV predominantly in terms of these two types of injury. Day-to-day embarrassments and humiliations, social rejection outside the jurisdiction of law, violence, or simply the fear of some future bad consequences—all may be more salient manifestations of social risk than losing a job or having a test result mishandled. Policy-makers and advocates have often tried to capture these generalized bad effects in the concept of "stigma," but that powerful concept may have suffered from overuse and imprecision. Despite a strong scholarly base (92,93), many people continue to use stigma as a synonym for "anything bad that happens because of HIV." Its complexity as a psychosocial phenomenon in interpersonal relationships and its relation to the social conflicts in a society that brings together the extremes of open homosexuality and reactionary religiosity in the same civic space have not sufficiently penetrated HIV research. Hence, we know far too little about how stigmas of drug use, sexuality, contagion, and even race influence health-related behavior (94).

Because we know so little about the influence of stigma on health-related behavior, it is difficult to assess the effectiveness of law as a remedy. Has the legal response decreased stigma? We do not know whether or to what extent legal protection against social risk has influenced the behavior of its objects. Has it addressed the problems people face and influenced their behavior in positive ways? Evidence is slim. People with HIV have filed thousands of discrimination complaints under the Americans with Disabilities Act, and they have done better than most other litigants (95). But the mere fact that generally only a minority of people who could resolve their problems with a lawsuit actually file the suit should point to the limits of law as a means of resolving disputes or protecting rights. It is reasonable to assume that protection against discrimination and breach of privacy would enhance the well-being of those who are protected, but the general effects may not be entirely positive. The price of protection is accepting the label of "disability" (96). Similarly, the right of privacy is the mirror image of the secrecy so central to the management of stigma (92).

Courts and legislatures exhibited a widespread willingness to extend legal protection to people with HIV, particularly during the first decade of the epidemic, but one cannot take for granted the stability of this protection. The Supreme Court reaffirmed *Arline*'s general approach and explicitly extended it to HIV in *Bragdon v. Abbott* (97). In general, though, the court has read the disability discrimination laws quite narrowly, and lower courts have issued many questionable decisions going against people with HIV, including decisions analyzing the "significant risk" issue in ways that seem a bit less rational and humane than *Ar-*

line contemplated (98,99). In the 1990s, legislatures were far more likely to narrow or repeal HIV privacy laws than to strengthen them.

Even if law remains in its present form, the experience with HIV raises the question of whether law alone is sufficient to deal with social risks. There are many social risks that law does not address: it is illegal for an employer to fire a person because he has AIDS, but it is not illegal for members of a church congregation or other social group to shun him; a woman abandoned by her husband because she has HIV has no discrimination claim. Even where law provides a remedy in theory, it may not be effective in practice, as many victims of domestic violence will attest (100). For many people, the eventual remedy the law promises may not look substantial enough to overcome the immediate fear of being harmed: for example, a person whose unwillingness to be tested arises from fear of losing job, benefits, and social support may not be reassured by the possibility of winning money damages at the end of several years of employment discrimination litigation (67). And for some people, law is a hostile or alien force that is either inaccessible or positively dangerous to encounter (101,102).

The limits of law as a way of addressing social risk and sensitivity to social risk as a psychological phenomenon together have at least one very important implication for prevention and clinical practice: public health workers and health-care providers can play a significant positive role in addressing social risk. Laws can help make the social environment more favorable to disease prevention, but it is just as important to find ways to help individuals better cope with both the perception and the threat of social risk (94). Health-care providers can do much more to address patients' perceptions of social risk than just warning them of the risks and informing them of the law in the course of informed consent or counseling discussions. Indeed, merely warning people that HIV testing can be socially risky may actually make the risk appear greater to patients than it really is, or it may cause the patients to worry about the risks when they otherwise are comfortable with testing (103). Telling people about legal protection may not be as reassuring as the provider assumes. Securing informed consent to run a risk, though important, is never a substitute for minimizing or eliminating the risk. Along with information, patients need help in addressing their perceived risks and making sensible choices about whether the risk of testing or partner notification or health care outweighs its benefits—help that counselors, case managers, and even physicians may often be able to provide—and which will usually be more accessible than help from the legal system (104).

The Health and Human Rights Framework

In recent years, human rights have profoundly influenced the field of public health. Scholars may reasonably inquire why a body of international law dating back to the mid-twentieth century would suddenly become part of public health discourse. The emphasis on individual rights and liberties that emerged in the AIDS pandemic later in the century provides an important part of the explanation. Civil libertarians turned to the language of human rights to defend persons living with HIV/AIDS from the threats of stigma and discrimination.

Scholars and practitioners came to see human rights as essential tools in the work of public health. In part, they were responding to the problem of social risk in public health, as we have already described (88). But their vision was broader. The late Jonathan Mann, who was the first head of the World Health Organization's Global Programme on AIDS, used the HIV pandemic as a departure point to advocate for the use of human rights in public health. He theorized that public health and human rights are complementary fields motivated by the paramount value of human well-being. He believed that people could not be healthy if governments did not respect their rights and dignity and engage in health policies guided by sound ethical values. Nor could people have their rights and dignity if they were not healthy (105,106,107). Mann and his colleagues thus went beyond the claim that law could serve public health by protecting those with and at risk of disease from social risks. They argued more broadly that the observance of human rights was, in essence, a determinant of health (107,108).

Mann's passion for health and human rights in the AIDS pandemic, and the broad intellectual and emotional appeal of human rights generally, profoundly influenced a generation of scholars, practitioners, and activists. It is now common, even fashionable, to use the discourse of public health and human rights as social commentary or as a tool of scholarly analysis. People in the fields of public health, law, and ethics collaborate much more often and express each other's language and ideas. The rhetoric of ethics and human rights is frequently applied to the theory and practice of public health.

The language of human rights is used within public health in different, but overlapping, ways that are important to distinguish (109). Legal scholars and practitioners use human rights to refer to a body of international law that originated in response to the egregious affronts to peace and human dignity committed during World War II. The main source of human rights law within the United Nations system is the International Bill of Human Rights comprising the United Nations Charter, the Universal Declaration of Human Rights (UDHR), and two International Covenants of Human Rights. Human rights are also protected under regional systems, including those in American, European, African, and Arab countries. Human rights law follows a set of internationally agreed rules specified in the text of treaties and other instruments, is informed by precedent, and is interpreted by tribunals and commissions. International human rights law seldom provides easy answers but struggles to define and enforce human rights in the context of the legitimate powers of governments and the needs of communities.

Ethicists use the language of human rights for related, but different, purposes. The fields of ethics and human rights share an abiding belief in the paramount importance of individual rights and interests, but beyond that their perspectives diverge. While human rights scholars stress the importance of treaty obligations, ethicists seldom refer to international law doctrine. While human rights scholars rely on text and precedent, ethicists employ philosophical reasoning and argumentation. When ethicists adopt the language of international human rights, therefore, there is bound to be a certain amount of confusion. For example, if ethicists claim that health care is a "human right," do they mean that a definable and enforceable right under international law exists, or simply that philosophical principles such as justice support this claim?

Finally, advocates, as well as the public, often use the language of human rights for its aspirational, or rhetorical, qualities. Major public health schools, such as the Johns Hopkins University and Harvard University, give their students a copy of the UDHR at commencement or offer special certificates in human rights. When "rights" language is invoked, it is intended to convey the fundamental importance of the claim. It expresses the idea that government should adhere to certain standards, or provide certain services, because it is right and just to do so. Human rights as a symbol commands reverence and respect. Used in this aspirational sense, human rights need not be supported by text, precedent, or reasoning; they are self-evident, and government's responsibility simply is to conform.

The field of human rights has much work to do if it is to contribute usefully to health policy analysis. On the doctrinal level, for example, human rights scholars and advocates have not clarified the meaning of the right to health. The conceptualization of health as a human right, and not simply a moral claim, suggests that states possess binding obligations to respect, defend, and promote that entitlement. Considerable disagreement, however, exists as to whether "health" is a meaningful, identifiable, operational, and enforceable right, or whether it is merely aspirational or rhetorical. A right to health that is too broadly defined lacks clear content and is less likely to have a meaningful effect. If health is, in WHO's words, truly "a state of complete physical, mental and social well-being," then it can never be achieved. Even if this definition were construed as a reasonable, as opposed to an absolute standard, it remains difficult to implement and is unlikely to be justiciable. Vast scholarship and litigation in international fora were required to define and enforce civil and political rights. Social and economic rights, notably the right to health, deserve the same rigorous and sustained attention (110). This is beginning to happen in international fora. For example, the United Nations Committee on Economic, Social, and Cultural Rights recently offered detailed guidance on the meaning of the right to health (111).

Similarly, the broader empirical claim that the observance of human rights, or other law-related conditions of a society, can be seen as causally-related to health is both promising and difficult to pursue. There is a growing recognition throughout the disciplines of public health that what are variously called "structural," "environmental," and "fundamental social" causes of disease must be more effectively identified and addressed if we are to make substantial improvements in our understanding of the real determinants of population health (112,113). Ranging from specific social policies to the overall distribution of socioeconomic status, these conditions influence health by constituting the physical and social context in which individuals and communities behave, defining options and influencing choices. It is plausible and consistent with our experience of public health law during the HIV epidemic to hypothesize that the observance of human rights, and the operation of laws that order civil society, may be among the social determinants of health, or may be among the important mechanisms through which fundamental social determinants of health, such as social cohesion, are converted into health outcomes (114). Pursuing the epidemiological role of law and human rights will be valuable for social epidemiology, given the often important role law plays in supporting social structures. It will also be difficult, however. For both lawyers and other public health professionals, it will entail carefully distinguishing between normative claims—such as "human rights are important" or "everyone has a right to health"—and empirical ones, such as "human rights are important *to health*" or "observing the right to health will produce healthier populations."

The health and human rights framework has succeeded in inspiring a new generation of public health lawyers and activists—and even some in the other disciplines of public health—to focus attention on the role of governments and legal systems in health. It has provided a new set of benchmarks in the form of rights and a vocabulary for demanding change. In this, the movement recalls earlier efforts in the history of public health, from the work of Engels and Virchow to the British Committee for the Study of Social Medicine (115). Like these earlier movements did, the health and human rights movement now faces the challenge of building an effective structure of advocacy and intervention on the foundation of social epidemiology. Whether it will succeed to the extent of Mann's hopes is an open question, but there is no question that the health and human rights perspective matters in public health work, and that its salience is the result, in large part, of the HIV/AIDS epidemic.

Conclusion

The emergence of HIV/AIDS was a deeply unsettling event in the United States. As it does in many other matters of social uncertainty and conflict in this country, the law provided a vocabulary, a forum, and a set of regulatory tools for social factions responding to the disease. Virtually every aspect of HIV prevention and treatment was at one time or another a matter of legislation or litigation. Public health law was once again front-page news, and a matter of day-to-day interest for public health professionals. This chapter has described the extraordinary range of legal developments sparked by the HIV epidemic, and how together they revived the field of public health law.

The question of what the changes in public health law related to HIV/AIDS mean for the future of public health is particularly pressing in the wake of September 11, 2001. The use of anthrax as a weapon of terror, and the fear of worse pathogens being unleashed, has presented public health with a challenge every bit as fundamental as (if quite different from) that posed by the emergence of HIV. Many of the same questions are presented: about the role of coercion, about the legal infrastructure of public health work, about the readiness of the public health workforce to exercise the authority it has. Have HIV/AIDS changed the questions we ask or the answers we give?

Despite the renewed interest in public health law resulting from the HIV epidemic, and despite period studies documenting the problems with the laws setting out public health authority, little was done to revise state public health law. The anthrax attack of fall 2001 found the same unraveling legal structure that the IOM had condemned in the 1980s and that legal scholars documented in the 1990s (13,14). Fortunately, the revival of interest in public health law had produced a corps of trained public health lawyers who quickly responded by drafting a model public health emergency statute, assisted by a large number of legal collaborators in academia and in state and federal health agencies (116). This legal readiness must be attributed to HIV/AIDS. Indeed, in a world in which each new health threat presents new and unique challenges, the lesson of HIV for public health law may be that "the readiness is all," as William Shakespeare stated in *Hamlet*.

Our experience with HIV/AIDS did not produce a total rejection of coercion in public health law. Health authorities continue to need the power to take coercive action in order to protect the public. For example, the deemphasis on coercion in HIV/AIDS control did not extend to the control of tuberculosis in the 1990s and is very likely to have no effect on the response to a bioterror attack. When the population is seriously threatened, few would quarrel with the maxim that "the health of the people is the supreme law." HIV/AIDS has, however, made us more conscious of the risk that public fear in the face of disease can lead to health measures that unnecessarily harm individual rights, and to stigma and discrimination that can actually harm public health. Public health law provides some check on the arbitrary use of state power against people thought to pose a health risk by requiring fair, transparent procedures and the presentation of evidence that coercion is justified. These requirements are not always a true check, procedures only being as sound as the people applying them, but they are still valuable compared to the alternative of no process and no standards.

At the same time, the idea that law's vocabulary of powers, duties, and rights provides a useful framework for analyzing problems of prevention and treatment, along with Mann's suggestion that human rights can inform the practice of public health, offers great promise as a means of integrating social epidemiology and social justice. At the population level, the most pressing public health right of individuals is not to be free from interference when they pose a significant risk, but to face fewer risks. A focus on the individual's right to be free from specific interference from society obscures the practical and moral obligation of society to collectively create the conditions in which individuals have healthy options. In this, the lessons of HIV/AIDS are transferable to conditions as diverse as low birthweight and hypertension.

HIV/AIDS has shown us that it is particularly important to build a broader base of empirical research on law's many roles in public health. In the past few years, there has been growing interest in and support for public health law research and training within public health. The future effectiveness of law as a tool of public health depends on the course of this trend, powered in large part by the HIV/AIDS epidemic.

Renewed interest in public health law has also pointed researchers to law as an important contributing cause of disease or as a mechanism through which other social determinants of disease are expressed in health outcomes. This reflects a recognition that law is not simply a set of rules, but a collection of rules, institutions, behaviors and attitudes deeply embedded in our social structure. This sort of analysis of law is challenging, both socially and methodologically, but it has great promise well beyond HIV. At the very least, it may help further the integration of the social science study of law into epidemiology and the behavioral sciences of public health. Over time, it may help lawyers, policy-makers, and others outside public health better understand how "non-health" policies like taxation and education and equal employment opportunity can have meaningful health consequences.

Perhaps the best measure of the impact of HIV on public health law is that one chapter can only scratch the surface of the changes and challenges this continuing epidemic has brought to the field. One leaves the topic with only two certainties for the future: that law can do much more to help assure the conditions in which people can be healthy, and that our experience with HIV/AIDS has given us a clearer vision of that future.

References

1. Gostin LO: *Public Health Law: Power, Duty, Restraint.* University of California Press, Berkeley, 2000.
2. *Jacobson v. Massachusetts*, 197 U.S. 11 (1905).
3. Gostin, LO: Traditional public health strategies. In Dalton HL, Burris S, and the Yale AIDS Law Project: *AIDS and the Law: A Guide for the Public.* Yale University Press, New Haven, 1987, pp. 47–65.
4. Burris S: Fear itself: AIDS, herpes and public health decisions. *Yale Law Policy Rev* 3: 479–518, 1985.

5. Grad FP: *The Public Health Law Manual*. American Public Health Association, New York, 1970.

6. Christoffel T: *Health and the Law: A Handbook for Health Professionals*. Free Press, New York, 1982.

7. Wing KR: *The Law and the Public's Health*. Health Administration Press, Ann Arbor, Mich., 1974.

8. Tobey JA: *Public Health Law: A Manual of Law for Sanitarians*, 2nd ed. Commonwealth Press, New York, 1939.

9. Parker L and Worthington RH: *The Law of Public Health and Safety, and the Powers and Duties of Boards of Health*. Bender, Albany, NY, 1892.

10. Cooley TM: *A Treatise on the Constitutional Limitation which Rest upon the Legislative Power of the States of the American Union*. Little, Brown, Boston, 1878.

11. Freund E: *The Police Power: Public Policy and Constitutional Rights*. Calaghan, Chicago, 1904.

12. Tiedeman CG: *A Treatise on the Limitations of Police Power in the United States*. F. H. Thomas Law Book, St. Louis, 1886.

13. Gostin LO, Burris S, and Lazzarini Z: The law and the public's health: a study of infectious disease law in the United States. *Columbia Law Rev* 99: 59–128, 1999.

14. Institute of Medicine: *The Future of Public Health*. National Academy Press, Washington DC, 1998.

15. Rosenberg CE: *The Cholera Years*, 2nd ed. University of Chicago Press, Chicago, 1987.

16. Rosenkrantz BG: *Public Health and the State: Changing Views in Massachusetts, 1842–1936*. Harvard University Press, Cambridge, 1972.

17. Ellis JH: *Yellow Fever and Public Health in the New South*. University Press of Kentucky, Lexington, 1992.

18. Fox DM: Social policy and city politics: tuberculosis reporting in New York, 1889–1900. *Bull Hist Med* 49: 169–194, 1975.

19. Brandt AM: *No Magic Bullet: A Social History of Venereal Disease in the United States since 1980*. Oxford University Press, New York, 1987.

20. *LaRocca v. Dalsheim*, 120 Misc. 2d 697, 467 N.Y.S. 2d 302 (1983).

21. Schwartz FAO and Schaffer FP: AIDS in the classroom. *Hofstra Law Rev* 14: 163–190, 1985.

22. Hermann DHJ: The development of AIDS federal civil rights law: anti-discrimination law protection of persons infected with human immunodeficiency virus. *Indiana Law Rev* 33: 783–861, 2000.

23. Buss, WG: Educating children with human immunodeficiency virus. In David Webber, Ed. *AIDS and the Law*, 2nd ed. Wiley, New York, 1992, p. 125.

24. Burris S: Prisons, law and public health: the case for a coordinated response to epidemic disease behind bars. *Miami Law Rev* 47: 291–335, 1992.

25. Herman DHJ and Burris S: Torts: private lawsuits about HIV. In Burris S, Dalton HL, and Miller JL (eds.): *AIDS Law Today: A New Guide for the Public*. Yale University Press, New Haven, 1993, pp. 334–364.

26. Dalton, HL: Criminal law. In Burris S, Dalton HL, and Miller JL (eds.): *AIDS Law Today: A New Guide for the Public*. Yale University Press, New Haven, 1993, pp. 242–262.

27. Banks, TL: Reproduction and parenting. In Burris S, Dalton HL, and Miller JL (eds.): *AIDS Law Today: A New Guide for the Public*. Yale University Press, New Haven, 1993, pp. 216–241.

28. Burris, S: Testing, disclosure and the right to privacy. In Burris S, Dalton HL, and Miller JL (eds.): *AIDS Law Today: A New Guide for the Public.* Yale University Press, New Haven, 1993, pp. 115–149.

29. Scherzer, M: Private insurance. In Burris S, Dalton HL, and Miller JL (eds.): *AIDS Law Today: A New Guide for the Public.* Yale University Press, New Haven, 1993, pp. 404–432.

30. Burris S: Dental discrimination against the HIV-infected: empirical data, law and public policy. *Yale J Regul* 13: 1–104. 1996.

31. Mandelker, DR: Housing issues. In Burris S, Dalton HL, and Miller JL (eds.): *AIDS Law Today: A New Guide for the Public.* Yale University Press, New Haven, 1993, pp. 319–333.

32. Dennis, DI: HIV screening and discrimination: the federal example. In Burris S, Dalton HL, and Miller JL (eds.): *AIDS Law Today: A New Guide for the Public.* Yale University Press, New Haven, 1993, pp. 187–215.

33. *New York Society of Surgeons v. Axelrod* 572 N.E. 2d 605 (N.Y. 1991).

34. Gostin LO, Porter L, Sandomire H, and the U.S. AIDS Litigation Project: *Objective Description of Trends in AIDS Litigation.* U.S. Government Printing Office and Kaiser Family Foundation, 1990; 2nd ed., United States Government Printing Office and Kaiser Family Foundation, 1993; 3rd ed., U.S. Government Printing Office and Kaiser Family Foundation, 1996.

35. Gostin LO, Webber DW, and the U.S. AIDS Litigation Project: HIV/AIDS in the courts in the 1990s, Part 1. *AIDS Public Policy* 12: 105–121, 1997.

36. Gostin LO, Webber DW, U.S. AIDS Litigation Project: HIV/AIDS in the courts in the 1990s, Part 2. *AIDS Public Policy* 13: 3–19, 1998.

37. Burris S: HIV-infected health care workers: the restoration of professional authority. *Arch Family Med* 5: 102–106, 1996.

38. Gostin LO: The AIDS litigation project: a national review of court and human rights commission decisions, Part I: the social impact of AIDS. *JAMA* 263: 1961–1972, 1990.

39. Gostin LO and Webber DW: HIV infection and AIDS in the public health and health care systems: the role of law and litigation. *JAMA* 279: 1108–1113, 1998.

40. *AIDS Litigation Reporter.* Andrews Publications, Wayne, PA, 1998–current.

41. Webber D (ed.): *AIDS and the Law.* Aspen Publishing, New York, 1987.

42. Aiken J and Musheno M: Why have-nots win in the HIV litigation arena: socio-legal dynamics of extreme cases. *Law Policy* 16: 267–297, 1994.

43. Kritzer H, Vidmar N, and Bogart W: To confront or not to confront: measuring claiming rates in discrimination grievances. *Law Soc Rev* 25: 875–887, 1991.

44. Weiler PC, et al.: *A Measure of Malpractice: Medical Injury, Malpractice Litigation, and Patient Compensation.* Harvard University Press, Cambridge, 1993.

45. Siegelman P and Donohue JJ: Studying the iceberg from its tip: a comparison of published and unpublished employment discrimination cases. *Law Soc Rev* 24: 1133–1170, 1990.

46. Voelker R: Will focus on terrorism overshadow the fight against AIDS? *JAMA* 286: 2081–2083, 2001.

47. Burris, S: Clinical decision making in the shadow of law. In Anderson JR and Barret B (eds.): *Ethics in HIV-Related Psychotherapy: Clinical Decision Making in Complex Cases.* American Psychological Association, Washington, DC, 2001, pp. 99–129.

48. State statutes dealing with HIV and AIDS: a comprehensive state-by-state summary. *Law Sexuality* 8: 1–530, 1998.

49. Gostin LO and Hodge JG: The "names debate": the case for national HIV reporting in the United States. *Albany Law Rev* 61: 679–743, 1998.

50. Kramer KM: A national epidemic, a national conversation, a national law: in support of unique identifier reporting for HIV surveillance. *J Contemp Health Law Policy* 16(1): 173–209, 1999.

51. Gostin LO, Ward JW, and Baker AC: National HIV case reporting for the United States: a defining moment in the history of the epidemic. *N Engl J Med* 337: 1162–1167, 1997.

52. Turnock BJ and Kelly CJ: Mandatory premarital testing for human immunodeficiency virus: the Illinois experience. *JAMA* 261: 3415–3418, 1989.

53. *T.E.P. v. Leavitt*, 840 F. Supp. 110 (D. Utah 1993).

54. American Bar Association AIDS Coordinating Committee: *Deregulation of Hypodermic Needles and Syringes as a Public Health Measure: A Report on Emerging Policy and Law in the United States.* American Bar Association, Washington, DC, 2001.

55. Burris, S: Education to reduce the spread of HIV. In Burris S, Dalton HL, and Miller JL (eds.): *AIDS Law Today: A New Guide for the Public.* Yale University Press, New Haven, 1993, pp. 82–114.

56. Gostin LO: A proposed national policy on health care workers living with HIV/AIDS and other blood-borne pathogens. *JAMA* 284: 1965–1970, 2000.

57. *Crime Control Act of 1990,* 42 U.S.C. § 3756(f) (1990).

58. Greenberg MD: AIDS, experimental drug approval, and the FDA new drug screening process. *NYU J Legis Public Policy* 3: 295–350, 1999–2000.

59. McGovern TM: *S.P. v. Sullivan*: The effort to broaden the social security administration's definition of AIDS. *Fordham Urban Law J* 21: 1083–1122, 1994.

60. 29 C.F.R. §§ 1910.1030 (1999).

61. Blankenship KM, Bray SJ, and Merson MH: Structural interventions in public health. *AIDS* 14: S11–21, 2000.

62. Bayer R and Fairchild-Carino A: AIDS and the limits of control: public health orders, quarantine, and recalcitrant behavior. *Am J Public Health* 83: 1471–1476, 1993.

63. Gottfried RN: Lessons from Chautauqua county. *Albany Law Rev* 61: 1079–1090, 1998.

64. Bobinski MA. Patients and providers in the courts: fractures in the Americans with Disabilities Act. *Albany Law Rev* 61: 785–830, 1998.

65. Gellert G, et al.: Managing the non-compliant HIV-infected individual: experiences from a local health department. *AIDS Public Policy* 8: 20–26, 1993.

66. Burris S: Legal Aspects of regulating bathhouses and sex clubs: cases from 1984–1995. In press.

67. Burris S: Driving the epidemic underground? A new look at law and the social risk of HIV testing. *AIDS Public Policy* 12: 66–78, 1997.

68. Bayer R: *Private Acts, Social Consequences: AIDS and the Politics of Public Health.* Free Press, New York, 1989.

69. Institute of Medicine, National Academy of Sciences: *Confronting AIDS: Directions for Public Health, Health Care, and Research.* National Academy Press, Washington, DC, 1986.

70. National Commissions on AIDS: *AIDS: An Expanding Tragedy.* Author, Washington, DC, 1993.

71. Office of the United Nations High Commissioner for Human Right and the Joint United Nations Programme on HIV/AIDS: *HIV/AIDS and Human Rights: International Guidelines.* Published by United Nations Geneva, 1998.

72. *School Board of Nassau County v. Arline*, 480 U.S. 273 (1987).

73. Gostin LO: The Americans with Disabilities Act and the corpus of anti-discrimination law: a force for change in the future of public health regulation. *Health Matrix: J Law-Med* 3: 89–104, 1993.

74. 29 C.F.R. § 16.02(r) (1997).

75. Bayer R: Public health policy and the AIDS epidemic: an end to HIV exceptionalism? *N Engl J Med* 324: 1500–1504, 1991

76. Burris S: Rationality review and the politics of public health. *Villanova Law Rev* 34: 933–982, 1989.

77. Novak WJ: *The People's Welfare: Law and Regulation in Nineteenth-Century America*. University of North Carolina Press, Chapel Hill, 1996.

78. Barron L: *Contagion and Confinement: Controlling Tuberculosis along the Skid Road*. Johns Hopkins University Press, Baltimore, 1998.

79. Burris S: Public health, "AIDS exceptionalism," and the law. *John Marshall Law Rev* 27: 251–272, 1994.

80. Bayer R, et al.: The dual epidemics of tuberculosis and AIDS: ethical and policy issues in screening and treatment. *Am J Public Health* 83: 649–654, 1993.

81. Gostin LO: The resurgent tuberculosis epidemic in the era of AIDS: reflections on public health, law, and society. *Maryland Law Rev* 54: 1–131, 1995.

82. Marks G, Burris S, and Peterman T: Reducing sexual transmission of HIV from those who know they are infected: the need for personal and collective responsibility. *AIDS* 13: 297–306, 1999.

83. Sunstein CR: Social norms and social roles. *Columbia Law Rev* 96: 903–968, 1996.

84. Lessig L: The regulation of social meaning. *Univ Chicago Law Rev* 62: 943–1043, 1995.

85. Koester SK: Copping, running, and paraphernalia laws: contextual and needle risk behavior among injection drug users in Denver. *Hum Organ* 53: 287–295, 1994.

86. Burris S: Law and the social risk of health care: lessons from HIV testing. *Albany Law Rev* 61: 831–895, 1998.

87. *Health Insurance Portability and Accountability Act of 1996*, Pub. L No. 104–191, 110 Stat. 1936.

88. Gostin LO and Lazzarini, Z: *Human Rights and Public Health in the AIDS Pandemic*. Oxford University Press, Oxford, 1997, pp. 27–30.

89. Burris S and Gostin LO: Genetic screening from a public health perspective: some lessons from the HIV experience. In Rothstein MA (ed.): *Genetic Secrets: Protecting Privacy and Confidentiality in the Genetic Era*. Yale University Press, New Haven, 1997, pp. 137–158.

90. Burris S, Gostin LO, and Tress D: Public health surveillance of genetic information: ethical and legal responses to social risk. In Khoury M, Burke W, and Thomson E (eds.): *Genetics and Public Health in the 21st Century: Using Genetic Information to Improve Health and Prevent Disease*. Oxford University Press, New York, 2000, pp. 527–546.

91. Burris S: Studying the legal management of HIV-related stigma. *Am Behav Sci* 42: 1229–1243, 1999.

92. Goffman E: *Stigma: Notes on the Management of Spoiled Identity*. Prentice Hall, Englewood Cliffs, NJ, 1963.

93. Herek G: AIDS and stigma. *Am Behav Sci* 42: 1106–1116, 1999.

94. Burris S: Disease stigma in public health law and research. Journal of Law, Medicine, and Ethics, in press.

95. Moss KM and Burris S: Unfunded mandate: an empirical study of the implementation of the Americans with Disabilities Act by the Equal Employment Opportunity Commission. *Kansas Law Rev* 50: 1–110, 2001.

96. Engel DM and Munger FW: Rights, remembrance and the reconciliation of difference. *Law Soc Rev* 30: 7–53, 1996.

97. *Bragdon v. Abbott*, 524 U.S. 624 (1998).

98. *Equal Employment Opportunity Commission v. Prevo's Family Market, Inc.*, 135 F.3d 1089 (6th Cir. 1998).

99. *Montalvo v. Radcliffe*, 167 F.3d 873 (4th Cir. 1999).

100. Bernstein, SE: Living under siege: do stalking laws protect domestic violence victims? *Cardozo Law Rev* 15: 525–567, 1993.

101. Ewick P and Silbey S: *The Common Place of Law.* University of Chicago Press, Chicago, 1998.

102. Musheno MC: Legal consciousness on the margins of society: struggles against stigmatization in the AIDS crisis. *Identities* 2: 102–122, 1995.

103. Scambler G: *Epilepsy.* London: Routledge 1989.

104. Burris, S: Surveillance, social risk and symbolism: framing the analysis for research and policy. *J AIDS* 25: S120–S127, 2000.

105. Mann J, Gostin LO, Gruskin S, et al.: Health and human rights. *J Health Hum Rights* 1: 6–23, 1994.

106. Mann JM, Gruskin S, Grodin MA, and Annas GJ (eds.): *Health and Human Rights: A Reader.* Routledge, New York, 1998.

107. Mann J: Medicine and public health, ethics and human rights. *Hastings Cent Rep* 27: 6–13, 1997.

108. Mann JM: Human rights and AIDS: the future of the pandemic. *J Marshall Law Rev* 30: 195–200, 1996.

109. Gostin LO: *Public Health Law and Ethics: A Reader.* Milbank Memorial Fund and University of California Press, New York, 2002.

110. Gostin LO: Human rights of persons with mental disabilities: the European Convention of Human Rights. *Int J Law Psychiatry* 23: 125–159, 2000.

111. *General Comment No. 14: The Right to the Highest Attainable Standard of Health,* E/C.12/2000/4, 4 July 2000.

112. Rose G: *The Strategy of Preventive Medicine.* Oxford University Press, Oxford, 1992, pp. 12–13.

113. Link, BG and Phelan J: Social conditions as fundamental causes of disease. *J Health Soc Behav* 38 (extra issue): 80–94, 1995.

114. Burris S, Kawachi I, and Sarat A: Integrating law and social epidemiology, *Journal of Law, Medicine, and Ethics,* in press.

115. Bayer RO, Oppenheimer GM, and Colgrove J: Health and human rights: old wine in new bottles? *Journal of Law, Medicine, and Ethics,* in press.

116. The Model State Emergency Health Powers Act. URL: http://www.publichealthlaw. net (February 4, 2002).

6

The Evolution of National Funding Policies for HIV Prevention and Treatment

JEFFREY LEVI

The usual version of the history of funding for HIV-related prevention and treatment programs is one that emphasizes the "exceptionalism" of HIV and the success of public health officials and advocates in obtaining funding for HIV-specific public health programs. Indeed, Figure 6–1 indicates, funding did increase dramatically in the first years of the epidemic for these categorical discretionary programs. But approaches to funding HIV prevention and care programs were not necessarily exceptional since they were patterned on preceding public health efforts to create and/or increase funding for specific health concerns. Such categorical programs, despite initial funding successes, often clash with each other for funding and tend to be poorly integrated with one another and the larger health-care delivery system.

This chapter will argue that special challenges posed by HIV gave policy-makers an opportunity to "think outside the box" in terms of the delivery and financing of prevention and care programs and their relationship to the underlying health-care delivery system. That did not occur to any large extent in the first two decades of the epidemic in the United States. Now, as the epidemic enters its third decade, U.S. policy-makers have begun to examine the structural challenges posed by their initial approaches taken in response to HIV in both the prevention and care services arenas. New models for providing prevention and care services are emerging beyond the traditional categorical approaches. However,

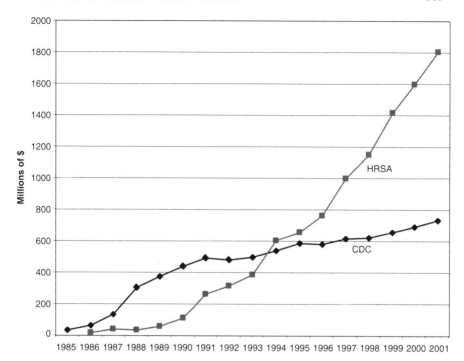

FIGURE 6–1. CDC and HRSA HIV/AIDS funding, 1985–2001. *Source*: Budget tables published annually by the Office of Management and Budget and the Department of Health and Human Services.

development of these new models is made more challenging by the fact that they must overcome established infrastructures. This chapter reviews the evolution of national funding policies for HIV prevention and care and highlights important lessons learned that may be applicable to other emerging public health challenges.

In responding to a new public health challenge (whether a newly recognized infectious disease such as HIV or, a new external threat such as bioterrorism), the immediate tendency is to create new programs separate from the rest of the public health system. In some instances this may be appropriate, but there are unintended costs involved in responding categorically. For example, multiple programs may be trying to reach the same target population—with duplicate dollars going toward the creation of redundant infrastructures in terms of program administration, data collection, and service delivery. Consider an analysis conducted in 2001 that revealed that 20 percent of people with HIV are already in the publicly funded Medicaid system when they get their HIV diagnosis (1). The same analysis revealed that these diagnoses are often late. Therefore, clients would have been better served by strengthening the programmatic relationships between federal and state public health programs and their Medicaid counterparts, rather than developing duplicate services to reach the same clients.

A particularly striking example of a missed opportunity to adopt an integrated approach is found in the delay in incorporating and supporting public health strategies into the existing health-care system. This reflects a common occurrence in public health: the belief that it can and should fix problems on its own. For example, the HIV care-related infrastructure supported with categorical funds through the Ryan White CARE Act was created separately from the rest of the categorical health-care safety net (i.e., the Community Health Centers program) and was not encouraged, until relatively recently, to create relationships with managed-care entities that serve people with HIV (2). And despite continued attempts to promote HIV prevention services in primary-care settings (3,4,5) abundant evidence exists that primary-care providers are not routinely providing prevention services to persons at high risk for HIV infection (6,7,8).

Indeed, an analysis of the effort to fund HIV-related prevention and treatment programs is a story of two worlds: the categorical programs created for people living with or at risk for HIV and the entitlement programs that were financing the bulk of the care and services received by people living with HIV. Public health officials and advocates, who focused their attention on the traditional categorical lines in the federal budget, paid little attention to the role of entitlement programs in delivering care and prevention services during the first fifteen years of the epidemic. For the first decade and a half, from a policy and programmatic perspective, the two worlds rarely intersected. The result was a diffusion of the vast political energy the HIV epidemic produced, which hurt public health in general and HIV programs in particular because of the constant need to justify funding rather than focusing on the substance of how to make the existing (though evolving) health-care system more responsive to public health in general and HIV in particular.

This chapter describes the following: the programs for HIV prevention and treatment services that are available for people living with HIV or at risk for HIV; the context of creating a public health response to HIV in terms of who has been affected by HIV, how those individuals relate to the health-care system, and how the evolving health-care system (particularly the growth in managed care) has affected public health's ability to reach and serve those individuals; an overview of the funding history of HIV-related treatment and prevention programs, both categorical and entitlement; the programmatic and bureaucratic impact of a disease-specific approach to HIV treatment and prevention; and the challenges and lessons for HIV and public health in general in moving toward an integrated approach to prevention and treatment that considers both categorical and health-care systems approaches—and how they should interrelate.

This chapter addresses the U.S. domestic response to the HIV epidemic and focuses on the central, publicly funded programs for HIV treatment and prevention. These are Medicaid, Medicare, the Ryan White CARE Act, and the Center for Disease Control and Prevention's grants to states, cities, and non-governmental organizations. There are several other public programs that address prevention and care needs (e.g., the grants from the Substance Abuse and Mental Health Services Administration), but they have relatively small budgets.

Public Programs for HIV

Medicaid is a federally established entitlement program jointly administered and funded with the states to finance the health-care of some poor Americans. Poverty alone does not make one eligible for Medicaid. Eligibility rules require an individual to be poor and in one of several classes of individuals: pregnant women, elderly, disabled, or children. Until 2000, when a handful of states sought permission to change eligibility criteria, most people living with HIV became eligible for Medicaid when their HIV became disabling (9). But for many poor women and children with HIV, their eligibility for Medicaid predated their HIV-caused disability. Income eligibility requirements are quite stringent. In most states the income of disabled people with HIV cannot be more than 75 percent of the federal poverty level, which in 2001 was $6,442 a year for an individual. Medicaid covers a very comprehensive set of treatment and preventive services, which are often far more extensive than those available in the private sector for HIV or any other condition.

Medicare is the federal insurance program most often associated with the elderly. In fact, certain disabled individuals are also eligible for Medicare coverage. Individuals who are disabled and eligible for Social Security Disability Income may become eligible for Medicare after a twenty-nine-month waiting period. While Medicare provides comprehensive inpatient and outpatient coverage, it does require copayments for services and does not (except in some managed-care plans) cover prescription drugs. For people with HIV, this last limitation is quite significant.

Congress passed the Ryan White Comprehensive AIDS Resources Emergency (CARE) Act of 1990 (RWCA) to help target discretionary dollars to cities and states to provide primary care and related support services to people living with HIV. The CARE Act was designed to relieve the added pressure AIDS had placed on the public health-care delivery infrastructure by emphasizing outpatient primary care and community-based support services that might reduce hospitalization time. These funds are distributed by the Health Resources and Services Administration for HIV-specific activities, separate from other "safety-net" programs that are designed to serve the uninsured and underserved, such as the community health centers program.

Also using discretionary dollars, the Centers for Disease Control and Prevention (CDC) provides grants to all state and some local health departments to support a variety of HIV-prevention-related services, including disease surveillance, primary prevention among those with HIV and at risk for HIV, and counseling and testing. In fiscal year 2001, of CDC's total HIV prevention appropriation of nearly $849 million, 46 percent (approximately $395 million), was awarded to state and local health departments to conduct HIV prevention activities. Non-governmental organizations, including community-based organizations funded directly with federal dollars, accounted for 20 percent of the appropriation ($166 million). A smaller portion of the annual budget funded school health activities (2.5 percent, or $21 million) (10).

Federal funding streams for HIV, STDs, and TB are separate, even though at the state level, these functions are often performed by the same staff. Varying degrees of program integration exist across public health departments for these three categorical activities. A survey conducted in 1997 by the Association of State and Territorial Health Officials demonstrated that most states are integrating these services at the administrative level (11).

The Demographics

Early in the epidemic, it was recognized that HIV disproportionately affects racial and ethnic minorities. HIV has also been described as a disease of poverty, since HIV transmission—especially as related to substance use—is associated with poverty in the United States. Many people with HIV started out poor and dependent on the public sector for the financing and the delivery of their health-care, or the costs associated with HIV care (and the inability to stay employed after an AIDS diagnosis in the early years, coupled with poor insurance protections) rendered an individual poor and dependent on the public sector as well.

Toward the end of the 1990s, with greater attention paid to the effect of HIV in minority communities, spurred by congressional and media attention, it is these demographics that drive a dependence on public-sector programs. People at risk for or infected with HIV are increasingly likely to be from racial or ethnic minority communities. Women, especially poor women of color, have some of the fastest rates of growth in HIV infection, followed by racial and ethnic minority men who have sex with men, injecting drug users, youth (particularly adolescents and young adults of color), and residents of inner-city urban areas (12). These same populations are more likely to be dependent on the public health-care financing and delivery system, especially Medicaid.

This dependence on the public sector is borne out by data from two studies supported by the federal government. The CDC Supplemental HIV/AIDS Surveillance (SHAS) study reported in 1997 that 83 percent of people with HIV or AIDS have no insurance or have their care financed by public programs such as Medicaid. In the SHAS sample, 75 percent of the people with HIV were unemployed (13). In the mid-1990s, the Agency for Health-care Policy Research

(AHCPR) funded the Health-care Services and Utilization Survey (HCSUS), which found that 68 percent of people living with HIV had no insurance or had their care financed through the Medicaid and Medicare programs (14).

The primary care services financed by Medicaid are relatively comprehensive. Medicaid also can finance prevention services and HIV counseling and testing for those at risk. Thus the Medicaid program should ideally be a focus of attention for program administrators and policy-makers who care about both HIV prevention and treatment services. Indeed, various data support the proposition that one can reach many people infected with HIV or from those populations at disproportionately high risk of infection through the Medicaid program:

- The U.S. Centers for Medicare and Medicaid Services, which runs the Medicaid program, estimates that 55 percent of adults living with an AIDS diagnosis (not HIV), are on Medicaid; 90 percent of children with AIDS are also on Medicaid (9).
- Twenty-nine percent of those with HIV or AIDS who are in regular care are on Medicaid only, and a higher percentage are dually eligible (14).
- One-third of poor women and 13 percent of near-poor women (i.e., 100 to 199 percent of poverty), regardless of HIV status, are on Medicaid (15).
- Medicaid pays for nearly 40 percent of all births in the United States (16).
- Twenty-one percent of all African Americans, regardless of HIV status, are on Medicaid (12); 43 percent of African Americans with HIV are on Medicaid only (14).
- Eighteen percent of Hispanics, regardless of HIV status, are on Medicaid (16), and 38 percent of Hispanics with HIV are on Medicaid only (14).
- Twenty percent of people with HIV are already on Medicaid when they receive their HIV diagnosis (1).

Entitlement Programs versus Categorical Programs

Medicaid is an entitlement program. If an individual meets the eligibility criteria, then that individual is guaranteed coverage under the program. As an entitlement program, funding is assured: spending automatically rises with the growth in enrollees. Unlike categorical or discretionary health programs (e.g., CDC prevention grants or HRSA Ryan White CARE Act grants), Medicaid is not subject to the vagaries of the annual federal budget appropriations cycle. If demand increases, so will funding. And demand has been growing over time for HIV-related services. Indeed, while most of the attention for HIV funding has been paid to the CARE Act and CDC funding for HIV prevention programs, Medicaid and Medicare have greatly outstripped spending on these discretionary programs (Figure 6–2).

These data highlight the importance of the Medicaid program as a means of reaching and serving both those living with HIV and at risk for HIV. Yet, in fact,

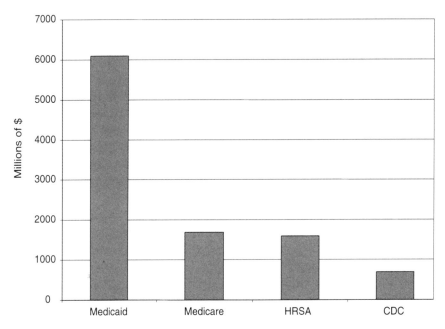

FIGURE 6–2. HIV care and prevention spending for year 2000. *Source*: Department of Health and Human Services budget tables.

the political attention of the AIDS community has been focused on creating and building the Ryan White CARE Act programs, and only in recent years has political energy been focused on the importance of the Medicaid program, and then only on Medicaid as a source of financing treatment rather than as a vehicle for supporting prevention services. The AIDS community's attention to Medicaid came about after the 1994 elections and the change in the control of Congress. Part of the new Republican majority's agenda was to convert Medicaid from an entitlement program (i.e., where all eligibles are guaranteed access) to a block grant as a "capped" entitlement (i.e., where a fixed amount of money would be available, thus potentially limiting the number of people eligible or the range of services that could be provided). This posed a potential threat to an important source of care financing for people living with HIV, and for the first time the AIDS community mobilized in support of Medicaid. Efforts to convert the Medicaid program have been blocked in the past; but with constant pressure on state budgets and recurring concerns about the cost of Medicaid to the federal government, this issue may arise again in some form.

More recently, the AIDS community's interest in Medicaid has focused on some of the deficiencies of the Medicaid program's eligibility criteria—namely, requiring a person with HIV to be disabled before becoming eligible, even as current research suggests that earlier treatment could prevent disability. For poor people with HIV, who cannot get on Medicaid until they are poor *and* disabled, this presents a "Catch-22" situation: the very treatments that might prevent their disability are inaccessible to them until they become disabled. Obviously, those eligible for Medicaid for non-HIV related reasons, such as pregnancy, might get access to early HIV intervention. Using demonstration authority under the Medicaid statute, some states are exploring options for expanding Medicaid eligibility to all poor individuals with HIV, regardless of disability status, on the argument that providing early treatment may be cost saving in the long run, if the need for more expensive disability-related care can be postponed or prevented altogether. At the time of this writing, the District of Columbia, Maine, and Massachusetts have received approval for such an expansion.

The HIV-related primary care services supported by the Ryan White CARE Act appear to have been established without due regard as to how the program could productively interact with the Medicaid program. Both the CARE Act and Medicaid cover primary-care services for people with HIV. However, the CARE Act also funds many supportive services such as social case management (an approach that goes beyond traditional medical case management to address the underlying social needs of persons with HIV disease) that Medicaid does not cover. Despite the requirements for a comprehensive planning process for spending most of the CARE Act's funds, a review of the early plans and guidances conducted by this author showed that minimal attention was paid to how the CARE Act would relate to the Medicaid program. Indeed, congressional pressure has inspired HRSA to take measures to enforce the legal requirement that CARE Act dollars be the "payer of last resort"—that no other payer, (Medicaid, Medicare, or private insurance) be available for this service (17). In reality, enforcement of this provision remains problematic (18). This reflects a failure of vision on the part of the creators and administrators of the CARE Act. By focusing on their "own" categorical program, they did not see the broader health-care system as the true core of safety net services for people living with HIV, with the CARE Act building infrastructure that wraps around and reinforces weaknesses (in services covered, in eligibility requirements, etc.) in that safety net.

In terms of HIV prevention, even less attention was paid to Medicaid and Medicare by policy-makers, except in the case of perinatal HIV transmission. As noted, 90 percent of children with AIDS are on Medicaid, and Medicaid pays for nearly 40 percent of all live births in the United States; thus it was hard to ignore Medicaid as a vehicle for ensuring access to treatments that prevent perinatal transmission of HIV. Preventing perinatal transmission of HIV by providing antiretroviral drugs to pregnant women with HIV is a traditional medical intervention. For nonclinical interventions such as community-based interventions to promote HIV testing or individual interventions to promote behavioral change by those with HIV or at risk for HIV, Medicaid was simply not on the radar screen of most public health officials during the first two decades of the epidemic: they did not see, or use, Medicaid as a vehicle for promoting and implementing broader HIV prevention efforts—this despite data showing that those who should be targeted for HIV counseling and testing and for prevention services could often be found in the Medicaid system and that many of the services provided as HIV prevention could be reimbursed under Medicaid.

It is perhaps not surprising that the attention of CARE Act administrators and HIV advocates to Medicaid was delayed, since they saw incredible growth in funding for their own programs. But federal HIV/AIDS spending varies greatly by category. Prevention funding has always been a "poor cousin" in the hierarchy of domestic HIV-related discretionary spending. Biomedical research has always received the highest level of funding and the most consistent growth in funding (about $2 billion in FY 2000), followed by the CARE Act (about $1.6 billion in FY 2000), with CDC's prevention programs (just under $700 million in FY 2000) always lagging behind, in terms of proportion of funding and growth rates. The majority of federal HIV/AIDS prevention funds (nearly 90 percent in fiscal year 2000), are appropriated to the CDC. Other federal agencies, including the Food and Drug Administration, the Indian Health Service, and the Substance Abuse and Mental Health Services Administration (SAMHSA) receive smaller amounts for HIV prevention activities. In addition to directly appropriated funds for HIV projects at SAMHSA, there is a set-aside for HIV early-intervention services in the Substance Abuse Block Grant for high-incidence states. Despite the significant role of substance use in HIV transmission and the growing evidence of co-morbidities influencing the mental health of individuals with HIV, SAMHSA has not, to date, played a leading role in HIV prevention efforts.

Neglect of entitlement programs as viable venues for public health work is not unique to HIV. But there is a special irony with HIV since one of the principles of effective prevention programming is to take the program to the individual. As the data presented earlier show, both those at risk for HIV and those with HIV are most likely to be served through the Medicaid system. But integrating HIV primary prevention into Medicaid poses at least three conceptual challenges. First, public health officials must come to see the primary-care system as a critical vehicle for undertaking community-based HIV prevention. Second, the administrators of the various state Medicaid programs have to recognize and accept their responsibility for integrating HIV prevention into what is essentially a primary-care system. And third, primary-care providers must have the training and the willingness to undertake prevention responsibilities.

Limitations of Medicaid

Although it is necessary to improve the system's ability to deliver and support HIV prevention and care, Medicaid alone will never be the entire solution to providing HIV treatment or prevention services for a variety of reasons. First, Medicaid's tight eligibility criteria, which require relatively extreme levels of poverty, combined with the requirement of meeting some other criterion (e.g., disability or pregnancy), will always limit the reach of a Medicaid-based effort. In the absence of a broad expansion of Medicaid, discretionary programs will still be needed to reach those populations not served by Medicaid but for whom services are needed.

Also, while Medicaid receives direction and a majority of its funding from the federal government, the tremendous discretion given to the states in the administration of this program, both in terms of determining eligibility and in identifying benefits provided, leaves an important role for discretionary programs to "level the playing field" across the nation. For instance, persons with HIV in one state could be eligible for a robust range of preventive and treatment services under Medicaid, but if they moved to another state with more stringent eligibility criteria, they might be totally ineligible for any services under Medicaid.

Currently, about 56 percent of all Medicaid beneficiaries are in managed care (19). As more and more states require their Medicaid beneficiaries to be part of managed-care arrangements, it becomes critical for the state Medicaid agencies, as purchasers, to define clearly for the managed-care organizations what their expectations are in the areas of HIV treatment and prevention (20). This shift in Medicaid purchasing toward managed care has had a serious fiscal impact on public health departments' ability to provide direct services to patients. In the past, if a service was covered by Medicaid, health departments could recoup some of their costs by seeking Medicaid reimbursement. Now, when a state moves to managed-care, if the health department's clinics are not part of the managed-care network, they lose a critical source of revenue. This is the case across many public health functions, including HIV and STDs (21).

In addition, Medicaid funds do not help providers create the infrastructure needed to establish appropriate service programs for people with HIV. CARE Act and CDC discretionary funds have been vital to the establishment of a network of community-based service providers. These providers often offer services not delivered in the traditional health-care delivery system (e.g., peer prevention counseling, social case management). Often funded because they have close ties to affected communities, their very community-based orientation could make it a challenge to integrate them and their services into a more traditional health-care delivery system.

Finally, in the case of HIV prevention, there is the challenge of ensuring that primary-care providers are adequately trained and compensated for providing HIV prevention services. Indeed, the medical training of primary-care providers often neglects critical prevention issues such as STDs and drug use, and the reimbursement schemes of insurers (public and private, fee-for-service and managed care) provide few incentives to offer comprehensive HIV prevention interventions.

An Inefficient Patchwork

Despite the complexities and challenges, the fact remains that efficient and effective HIV treatment and prevention interventions must be designed with entitlement and discretionary programs simultaneously in mind. The current system of funding HIV care and prevention services is a complex web of programs and funding streams that pose a significant challenge to individuals seeking access to appropriate prevention and treatment services and to local service providers who are trying to provide a comprehensive and "seamless" continuum of services to their clients. Figure 6–3 shows the great variety of federal programs for HIV-related prevention and treatment. Given this heterogeneous mix, program administrators and service providers are challenged to bring together a range of programs with different eligibility criteria, coverage requirements, application and reporting procedures, to form a continuum of services for persons at high risk of acquiring HIV and those already infected with the virus. (Figure 6–3 actually underestimates the number of funding streams a provider might need to balance, as within Titles I and II of the CARE Act, for example, a jurisdiction may issue multiple requests for proposals.) This complex array of programming not only makes life more difficult for the clients and service providers but also creates inefficiencies, simply by requiring so many different layers of administrative support and oversight. For example, if we limit ourselves to just public treatment-related resources (putting prevention to the side for the moment, because prevention funds serve more than people with HIV), we will find from the following two tables that, in fact, there is a very high level of resources available on a per capita basis for HIV service provision. (See the following discussion on the relationship to the actual cost of care.)

Despite this significant investment in publicly funded HIV care, many people with HIV are not in care, either because they are unaware that they are infected or they have not entered the care system for one reason or another. The CDC estimates that between 650,000 and 900,000 Americans have HIV infection, of whom about 500,000 know their status (22). The HCSUS estimates that only 350,000 people living with HIV are in care (14). Ideally, all 500,000 who know

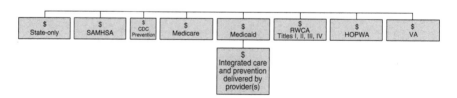

Figure 6–3. HIV funding streams for HIV-related treatment and prevention services. HOPWA, Housing Opportunities for People with AIDS; RWCA, Ryan White CARE Act; SAMHSA, Substance Abuse and Mental Health Services Administration; VA, Veterans Administration.

their status should be in care, even if they decide to delay treatment. In turn, aggressive outreach should be undertaken, targeting individuals who are infected but who have not yet been tested.

With a public investment of $10.6 billion in FY 2000 for HIV treatment and care services (Table 6–1), the question arises as to whether there are sufficient funds to provide appropriate care for all people living with HIV in the United States who might be dependent on the public sector. Given the earlier discussion of state-by-state variability in Medicaid and other programs, it is critical to remember that *national estimates may not necessarily reflect the reality in a given jurisdiction*. National figures can only paint a broad picture of the challenges associated with financing HIV-related care at the state and local level. That much said, Table 6–2 illustrates estimates of total public financing available for HIV-related care, if distributed evenly across the country. These estimates assume that 85 percent of all people with HIV would be totally dependent on the public sector, which is higher than most studies show. Per capita funding estimates are calculated using the midpoint of the CDC's estimate for all people living with HIV infection, all people who know their status, and all who are in care.

Based on current estimates of the annual cost of care for treating HIV, these resources should be sufficient to provide a full set of care services for people liv-

TABLE 6–1. Estimates of Public Spending on HIV-Related Care (FY 2000)

SOURCE	$ BILLION
Federal Resources	
Medicaid	3.3
Medicare	1.7
Ryan White CARE Act	1.6
SAMHSA	0.1
Veterans Administration	0.5
Housing Opportunities for People with AIDS	0.2
Total Federal Resources	**7.4**
State Resources	
Medicaid match	2.8
Discretionary ADAP spending	0.1
Estimated additional state-only spending	0.3
Total State Resources	**3.2**
Total Federal and State Resources	***10.6***

Sources: Estimated additional state-only spending based on FY 1996 reports submitted by the states to HRSA; state ADAP spending is for FY 2000 from National Alliance for State and Territorial AIDS Directors *National ADAP Monitoring Project Annual Report*, March 2001; Medicaid spending is from Centers for Medicare and Medicaid Services, Office of the Actuary; all other figures are from Kaiser Family Foundation, *Federal HIV/AIDS Spending: A Budget Chartbook*, 2000.

ADAP, AIDS Drug Assistance Programs.

TABLE 6–2. Estimated Public Funding Available per Person with HIV for Care Services

POPULATION	FY 2000 PER CAPITA $
All HIV+	$16,147
(775,000 × 85% = 658,750)	
All HIV+ who know status	$25,028
(500,000 × 85% = 425,000)	
All HIV+ in care	$35,755
(350,000 × 85% = 297,500)	

The estimates assume 85% dependence on the public sector. Number of HIV positives is midpoint of the CDC's estimate. Other estimates of the number of HIV positives who do not know their status are lower*; by using this larger estimate, a more conservative figure is derived for the amount of money available on a per capita basis.

*Estimates from Centers for Disease Control and Prevention, National HIV Testing Day at CDC-Funded HIV Counseling, Testing, and Referral Sites—United States, 1994–1998. *Morb Mortal Wkly Rep* 49: 529–532, 2000.

ing with HIV who know their status. One model estimates the range of treatment costs in the United States to be from $4,829 a year for those with early-stage HIV and who are not receiving drug therapy to $31,308 per year for persons with late-stage AIDS who are receiving drug therapy (23). Thus, on average, it appears that sufficient resources to care for all HIV-infected individuals in the United States should be available.

Despite the seeming sufficiency of funds to pay for the care of indigent HIV-infected individuals in the United States, anecdotal reports indicate that many are going without care. In a recent HRSA-sponsored national study of providers receiving CARE Act funds, 57 percent reported financial barriers to participation in the CARE Act (24). Over one-half (52 percent) of clinical providers, 56 percent of case management providers, and 55 percent of other social support providers reported that RWCA funds are "somewhat to very difficult" to obtain. Among providers experiencing financial barriers, 21 percent reported having insufficient funds to meet the demand for care. Lack of funds and limited capacity impede CARE Act providers from actively undertaking efforts to identify untreated HIV-infected individuals. In the cited study, fewer than one-half (43 percent) of clinical providers and 51 percent of case management and social support agencies reported providing outreach services (24).

How can these findings be explained? Several factors are likely working in concert. First, many programs that finance care for people living with HIV have multiple administrative structures at the national and state levels. Most CARE Act programs, for example, rely on multiple funding streams to support their programs (24). This complex infrastructure, while permitting providers to patch together appropriate treatment and care services for persons with HIV also creates inefficiencies and added administrative costs.

Second, Medicaid and Medicare eligibility criteria generally restrict enroll-ment of persons living with HIV until late in their disease progression. As a re-sult, HIV-infected persons continue to enter the HIV care system at advanced stages of disease when health-care costs are highest. Earlier access to care fi-nancing and HAART therapy through enrollment prior to disability, while pos-sibly a more cost-effective approach, is not permitted under current law.

Third, there is an uneven distribution of resources available across the coun-try. For example, in an HRSA-sponsored study of CARE Act providers, sub-stantial differences in the mix of clinical and social services were identified within communities, states, and regions (24). In some rural communities, only case man-agement or primary-care services were provided; in other communities, a wide array of clinical, ancillary medical care, substance abuse and mental health treat-ment, housing, case management, and social support services were funded. In some communities CARE Act providers report being denied cost of living in-creases for their staff or a chronic lack of additional funds to expand services. Ironically, some of these providers are located in areas contiguous to commu-nities that have received large increases in CARE Act funds that are being used to establish new programs or support new contractors (24). And despite a heavy infusion of new funds in recent years for AIDS Drug Assistance Programs (ADAP), several states continue to experience shortfalls in funds before the end of their fiscal year. These shortfalls have resulted in institution of narrow eligi-bility criteria, enrollment limits, waiting lists, or limited coverage for HAART and other drugs used in the treatment of HIV disease (25). While differences in the level of CARE Act funds is one contributing factor driving these geographic disparities, other forces such as the level of state funds dedicated to HIV care and the scope of Medicaid eligibility and coverage have also been important in-fluences.

Fourth, methods for distributing and monitoring CARE Act funds have intro-duced inefficiencies and administrative and financial barriers for providers. CARE Act providers report that procurement, grants management, and reporting sys-tems are burdensome, unnecessary, and unreasonable. Grant making and reim-bursement mechanisms have also been identified as being significantly prob-lematic. Of particular concern is the effect of administrative caps on the ability of programs to meet their increasing administrative and infrastructure develop-ment demands (24).

Implications for Other Public Health Efforts

The conclusion of this analysis is not that there are too many resources available for treating HIV, but that these resources, if better managed, could serve more people and facilitate the integration of primary HIV prevention services into the mix. The American response to HIV/AIDS has not paid adequate attention to the underlying system of financing and delivery of health-care in the United States, especially the poverty-based health-care system in which those who are in need of HIV prevention and treatment services are often found. Indeed, an important caution that can be drawn from the HIV experience with funding treatment and prevention programs is that, while it is possible to create wonderful, perhaps even elegant new responses to each disease, the result is not necessarily a more rational or more functional system.

Four basic lessons derived from the HIV/AIDS funding experience can be of benefit to future generations of policy-makers as they grapple with the challenges of funding emerging and recurrent public health problems.

First, policy-makers must take advantage of the data that the public health and other medical systems collect to drive the design and implementation of interventions and funding policies. As discussed here, this was not always done in the case of HIV, and the result has been missed opportunities to intervene with those at risk for HIV and to diagnose and treat those already infected. Too often, public health officials analyze (or collect) only the data related to morbidity and mortality and ignore useful data about how target populations are already interfacing with other components of the health-care delivery system.

Second, public health planners must think of the entire health-care system, not just the much smaller universe of public health–specific programs, as part of its armamentarium in responding to a public health emergency. In so doing, they must also take into account the evolving nature of that health-care delivery system. In the current climate, this means more and more managing of care by third-party payers, with limits on access and reimbursement to public health providers. Planners must actively strive to integrate public health interventions into the existing health-care delivery system, which requires a reconceptualization of how population-based interventions should be merged into an individual-based health-care system. While this poses both scientific and operational challenges, such integration is essential if public health interventions are to be brought to those who most need them.

Third, the design and implementation of *discretionary* public health programs must occur with conscious attention to the underlying health-care delivery system, especially the poverty-based Medicaid system. This will permit the targeting of discretionary funds to those populations outside the health-care delivery system and to those interventions that cannot be easily incorporated into existing health-care delivery systems.

Fourth, and perhaps most important, the HIV/AIDS funding experience has shown that policy-makers responsible for health programs of all kinds must find common philosophical ground in order to accept the integration of population-based public health approaches within the individual-oriented health-care delivery system. Making such integration a reality will entail removal of the countless administrative and procedural barriers that work against cooperative efforts among categorical and entitlement programs.

References

1. Levi J, Kates J, Neal J, Gallagher K: Targeting HIV prevention services for people with HIV and at risk for HIV based on care financing mechanism. Paper presented at the 2001 National HIV Prevention Conference, Atlanta, Georgia, August 13, 2001.
2. As part of the Special Projects of National Significance, the Health Resources and Services Administration is supporting the Center for Integrated HIV Care Networks, which is working with community-based organizations preparing to provide HIV care and social services in a managed care environment. The Center is housed at the George Washington University Center for Health Services Research and Policy. URL: www.gwhealthpolicy.org.
3. Gerber AR, Valdiserri RO, Holtgrave DR, et al.: Prevention services guidelines for primary care clinicians caring for adults and adolescents infected with the Human Immunodeficiency Virus. *Archives of Family Medicine* 2(9): 969–979, 1993.
4. Horsburgh CR, Douglas JM, and LaForce M: Preventive strategies in sexually transmitted diseases for the primary care physician. *JAMA* 258: 814–821, 1987.
5. American Medical Association: *A Physician Guide to HIV Prevention.* AMA, Chicago, 1996.
6. Boekeloo BO, Marx ES, Kral AH, et al.: Frequency and thoroughness of STD/HIV risk assessment by physicians in a high-risk metropolitan area. *Am J Public Health* 81: 1645–1648, 1991.
7. Green S and del Rio C: HIV pretest and postest counseling: still missing from medical school curriculum. *Arch Intern Med* 160:3326, 2000.
8. Schuster MA, Bell RM, Petersen LP, and Kanouse DE: Communication between adolescents and physicians about sexual behavior and risk prevention. *Arch Pediatr Adolesc Med* 150: 906–913, 1996.
9. Kaiser Family Foundation. *Medicaid's Role for Persons with HIV/AIDS.* Fact Sheet. Menlo Park, CA: Kaiser Family Foundation, October 2000.
10. Personal communication, Ron Valdiserri, Deputy Director, National Center for HIV, STD, TB Prevention, February 2002.
11. Association of State and Territorial Health Officials: *HIV/AIDS, STD, and TB Prevention Program Integration Survey of State Health Agencies.* Washington, DC, December 1997.
12. Centers for Disease Control and Prevention: *HIV Prevention Strategic Plan through 2005.* URL: http://www.cdc.gov/hiv/pubs/prev-strat-plan.pdf (January 2001), p. 7.
13. Nakashima AK: Who will pay for HIV treatment? Health insurance status of HIV-infected persons. *Proceedings of the 1997 Infectious Diseases Society of American.* Abstract 293. The SHAS study drew respondents primarily from public health clinics; thus it may overestimate the number of uninsured or unemployed individuals.
14. Bozzette S, et al.: The care of UV-infected adults in the United States: Results from the HIV cost and services utilization study. *N Engl J of Med* 339(26): 1897–1904, 1998.
15. Kaiser Family Foundation. *Medicaid's Role for Women.* Fact Sheet. Menlo Park, CA: Kaiser Family Foundation, November 2000.
16. Kaiser Commission on Medicaid and the Uninsured: *Medicaid Overview Briefing*

Charts. Menlo Park, CA: Kaiser Family Foundation, April 2001. URL: http://www.kff. org/content/2001/2244/2244.pdf.

17. See Ryan White CARE Act Amendments of 2000, Public Law 106-345.

18. Levi J., Hidalgo J, and Wyatt S: The impact of state-by-state variability in entitlement programs on the Ryan White CARE Act. In Ryan C (ed.): *Directions in HIV Service Delivery and Care: A Policy Brief*. Rockville, MD: Health Resources and Services Administration, vol. 2, pp. 15–20.

19. Health Care Financing Administration: *Managed Care Trends*. URL: http://www.hcfa. gov/medicaid/trends00.htm.

20. For an example of how such standards might be incorporated in a purchasing agreement, see the Center for Health Services Research and Policy: *Sample Purchasing Specifications for HIV Infection, AIDS, and HIV-Related Conditions*. George Washington University School of Public Health and Health Services. URL: www.gwu.edu/~chsrp.

21. Rosenbaum S, Mauery R, Blake S, and Wehr E: *Public Health in a Changing Health-Care System: Linkages between Public Health Agencies and Managed Care Organizations in the Treatment and Prevention of Sexually Transmitted Diseases*. Menlo Park, CA: Kaiser Family Foundation, 2000.

22. Centers for Disease Control and Prevention: Recent HIV/AIDS treatment advances and the implications for prevention. URL: www.cdc.gov/nchstp/hiv_aids/pubs/facts/ treatmnt.htm.

23. Kahn JG, Haile B, Kates J, and Chang S: The health and federal budgetary effects of increasing access to antiretroviral medications for HIV by expanding Medicaid. *Am J Public Health* 91: 1464–1473, 2001.

24. Hidalgo J, Rawlings MK, and Lewis R: *Participation of Racial and Ethnic Minority Providers in Clinical and Social Support Services Funded by the Ryan White CARE Act*. Annapolis: Positive Outcomes, Inc., 1999.

25. Doyle A, et al.: *National ADAP Monitoring Project Annual Report, March 2000*. National Alliance of State and Territorial AIDS Directors and AIDS Treatment Data Network, 2000.

7

AIDS and the Making of an Ethics of Public Health

RONALD BAYER

It was against the backdrop of a history of research abuse that contemporary bioethics took shape in the 1960s and 1970s (1). The fundamental thrust of the new perspective was to reconceptualize the balance of power between doctors and their patients and researchers and their subjects. In charting the course of the new bioethics, physicians, philosophers, theologians, lawyers, and social scientists drew on the legacy of largely ineffective efforts to impose constraints on research involving human subjects and the history of legal and professional norms that gave recognition to the principle that competent adults should determine if and when they would undergo medical interventions (2). The new efforts were indelibly marked by the broad struggle for rights of the poor and the socially and culturally disempowered that marked the era. As a consequence, bioethics was informed by the profound influence of individualism in American social life. As it targeted the practice of medicine and the conduct of research, bioethics gave pride of place to the concept of autonomy. Paternalism in all its guises was the subject of withering criticism.

But the bioethical challenge entailed something in addition to a set of substantive positions. Just as significant, it represented a challenge to the view that the central decisions of medicine were technical, founded on professional expertise. Instead, bioethics sought to underscore the underlying value dimension of such decisions. And in the face of conflicts about such values, decision mak-

ing required a more egalitarian posture, one that acknowledged the morally relevant basis of patient choice. Bioethics thus shared a radical dimension with many
of the activist movements of the 1960s and 1970s.

Despite its potentially far-reaching implications, however, what is so striking
about the bioethics that took hold in the United States was its almost singular focus on the challenges of the clinical and research encounter. Scant attention was
accorded to the public health. To be sure there were exceptions—some discussion of justice and access to health care, and of the questions posed by the policy implications of the behavioral association with chronic disease—but they only
served to underscore the relatively narrow range of issues that animated discussion within bioethics, which was seized by the dramatic developments in bio-
medicine.

Hence there was no sustained effort to consider the inherent dilemmas posed
by an enterprise that took the well-being of populations as its starting point, and
whose history was marked by the use of coercive interventions and a remarkable
paternalism. Were the strictures against paternalism in the dyadic context of the
clinical encounter appropriate to public health? How were the rights of the individual to be balanced against collective needs? These issues hardly merited attention. And so there was no occasion to confront the question of whether an
ethics grounded in individualism could prove productive as a guide to public policy that sought to advance the goals of health promotion and disease prevention
on a collective scale.

It would take the AIDS epidemic to provide the occasion for an extended encounter between bioethics and public health. What ethicists brought to the emerging challenge of AIDS in the early and mid-1980s was both an approach that
would move them to examine the underlying moral conflicts that characterized
the practice of public health and a set of moral convictions that placed the right
of the individual at center stage. It was a perspective that was compatible with
the fundamental shift that had begun to occur in the broad social and constitutional context within which public health functioned. The Supreme Court had developed a remarkable jurisprudence of privacy (3), linked to reproductive rights,
and had underscored the importance of protecting the procedural rights of individuals who were threatened with restrictions or deprivations of liberty. This was,
then, an era very different from that which permitted a legal treatise to assert in
the early part of the twentieth century that before public health "all constitutionally guaranteed rights must give way" (4), a perspective that could still find
expression in a California court decision of 1966 which declared that "health regulations enacted by the state under its police powers and providing even drastic
measures for the elimination of disease . . . in a general way are not affected by
constitutional provisions of the state of national governments (5).

In the course of the encounter between bioethics and AIDS, the substantive
commitment to the rights of the individual—to privacy, to the claim to be free

of unconsented medical interventions, to freedom from coercive paternalistic interventions—would serve as a critical element in the making of public health policy, especially in the epidemic's early years. As important, the encounter would ultimately serve as a catalyst for the development of an ethics of public health.

AIDS Exceptionalism: Testing, Reporting, and Partner Notification

In the early and mid-1980s, at the outset of the American encounter with AIDS, it was necessary to face a set of fundamental questions: Did the history of responses to lethal infectious diseases provide lessons about how best to contain the spread of HIV? Should the policies developed to control sexually transmitted diseases or other communicable conditions be applied to AIDS? If AIDS were not to be so treated, what would justify such differential policies?

To understand the importance of these questions, it is necessary to recall that conventional approaches to public health threats typically provided a warrant, when deemed appropriate, for mandating compulsory examination and screening, thus breaching the confidentiality of the clinical relationship by reporting to public health registries the names of those diagnosed with "dangerous diseases," imposing treatment, and, in the most extreme cases, confining persons through the power of quarantine. To be sure, many aspects of this public health tradition, forged at the outset of the twentieth century, had been modulated over the decades, in part because of changes in the patterns of morbidity and mortality.

Nevertheless, it was the specter of the historically coercive aspects of the public health tradition that most concerned proponents of civil liberties and advocates of gay rights and bioethics as they considered the potential direction of public health policy in the presence of AIDS, a disease that so disproportionately affected disfavored groups: gay men, drug users, the poor in minority communities. Although there were some public health traditionalists in the United States who pressed to have AIDS and HIV infection brought under the broad statutory provisions established to control the spread of sexually transmitted and other communicable diseases, they were in the distinct minority. In place of the conventional approach to public health threats, there emerged an alternative view— broadly defined as exceptionalist (6)—that took as its starting point the need to craft policies that were persuasive rather than coercive and that viewed the protection of the rights of those who were infected as integral rather than as antagonistic to the goals of disease prevention. For those who advanced this new perspective, privacy and confidentiality were to be accorded great importance. The goal was to avoid, at all costs, measures and practices that might be counterproductive, that might "drive the epidemic underground" by inspiring fear and distrust rather than by fostering engagement between public health officials and those most at risk. How the exceptionalist perspective with its commitment to noncoercive approaches to HIV affected policy is most clearly illustrated in the debates over HIV testing, reporting of HV, and partner notification efforts. In each of these arenas, the perspective of bioethics assumed a central, albeit differing, role.

From the moment of its introduction in 1985, the HIV test became the subject of intense debate. Fear that those identified as having HIV might be subject to discrimination and stigma; concern about how the diagnosis of HIV infection, in the absence of effective therapy, could produce unbearable psychological burdens; and a belief that testing had little to do with behavioral change—all led AIDS activists generally, and gay leaders specifically, to adopt a posture of hostility or skepticism regarding the test. Alternatively, many public health officials believed that the identification of infected persons could play a crucial role in fostering behavioral change. Out of their confrontations emerged a broad consensus that, except in a few well-defined circumstances, people should be tested only with their informed, voluntary, and specific consent (7).

In one of the first major statements on the ethical challenges posed by the AIDS epidemic, a group organized under the aegis of the Hastings Center, then among the preeminent organizations studying the ethical challenges of medicine, wrote the following in the *Journal of the American Medical Association*:

We believe that the greatest hope for stopping the spread of HIV infection lies in the voluntary cooperation of those at higher risk—their willingness to undergo testing and to alter their personal behavior and goals in the interests of the community. But we can expect this voluntary cooperation—in some cases sacrifice—only if the legitimate interests of these groups and individuals in being protected from discrimination are heeded by legislators, professionals, and the public. (8)

A group working out of the Johns Hopkins School of Public Health struck a similar posture when addressing the ethical issue of mandatory screening of pregnant women for HIV infection. The group concluded: "We reject the implementation of counseling and screening policies that interfere with women's reproductive freedom, or that result in the unfair stigmatization of vulnerable groups" (9). For reasons having to do with ethical and pragmatic concerns, the Centers for Disease Control and Prevention also embraced voluntary testing (10).

Much of the early ethical discussion of HIV testing occurred in the context of extreme therapeutic limits. As a result of clinical developments—the belief that treatment with zidovudine could delay the onset of symptomatic AIDS and the recognition of the importance of primary prophylaxis against *Pneumocystis carinii* pneumonia—by 1990, the medical significance of identifying those with early HIV disease had become clear. Consequently, the clinical and political context—involving a wide range of constituencies—of the debate about testing underwent a fundamental change (8). Gay organizations began to urge homosexual and bisexual men to have their antibody status determined under confidential or anonymous conditions. Physicians pressed for AIDS to be incorporated into the medical mainstream and for the HIV-antibody test to be treated like other blood tests—that is, given with the presumed consent of the patient. In the face of such pressure, those committed to the protection of the rights of the infected (among them the bioethicists who had been drawn to AIDS) continued to insist that testing only occur with specific informed consent. Whatever, in fact, occurred in the context of clinical settings, public policy at the federal and state level continued to reflect a commitment to the voluntaristic premise of the exceptionalist perspective and the enduring influence of the ethical underpinnings first enunciated in the mid-1980s when medicine was all but impotent.

Nevertheless, pressure to shift the paradigm of testing away from the exacting standard of informed consent continued to mount. It was especially pronounced in the case of pregnant women and newborns (11). Diagnostic progress was to make it possible to determine whether HIV-positive newborns were truly infected soon after birth, and the improved prospects of clinical management were to make such determinations for infected infants appear all the more critical. So it is not surprising that pediatricians became increasingly impatient with the strict regimen of explicit and specific consent that surrounded the testing of newborns for HIV (12), all the more so because routine and unconsented testing of newborns for inborn errors of metabolism such as phenylketonuria was mandated in virtually every state and had provoked little by way of ethical objection.

In late spring 1993, New York State, which together with California had pioneered the enactment of stringent informed consent requirements for HIV testing, seriously considered legislation that would have mandated the screening of newborns for HIV infection. When that legislation ultimately passed in 1996 (13), it provoked a cry of outrage from the advocates of women's rights and other defenders of exceptionalism. Ironically, the passage of a mandatory newborn testing statute occurred when interest had already begun to shift to the question of screening pregnant women. That shift had occurred in early 1994 as the result of the finding that the administration of zidovudine during pregnancy could reduce the rate of vertical transmission by two-thirds (14).

In the aftermath of that finding, pressure mounted to ensure that infected women were identified early in pregnancy. Although advocates on behalf of women's interests fought hard to preserve the right of pregnant women to undergo HIV testing only after specific informed consent, the prospect of saving newborns from HIV infection provided the foundation for an assault on that posture (15). In June 1996, the American Medical Association's House of Delegates passed a resolution calling for mandatory testing of pregnant women. Commenting on that decision, a past president of the association said, "The Association opposed testing early on because society had little to offer victims of HIV other than discrimination. But now that we can offer treatment and alter the course of the disease, and hopefully prevent it in the unborn child, we can embrace a more scientifically oriented position that might benefit all" (16). Even the Institute of Medicine, which early in the epidemic had opposed testing policies that abrogated the privacy rights of pregnant women, was by the end of the 1990s to endorse routine testing on the basis of an informed right of refusal, a much less exacting standard than specific informed consent (17).

The willingness to consider mandatory testing of newborns and pregnant women was eased by existing conventions that provided a warrant for prenatal and postnatal screening dictated by the interest of children. In other contexts, the retreat from the exceptionalism of the epidemic's early years—with its stress on an exacting standard of specific informed consent with pretest counseling—and the waning influence of the principles first put forward by ethicists, has taken the form of efforts to integrate HIV testing into clinical practice where standards of presumed consent prevail. Strikingly, however, when in 1999 the CDC proposed, as one of several options, a relaxation of the standard of specific informed consent for HIV testing in populations other than pregnant women, it provoked sharp opposition from those constituencies that had helped to shape the voluntaristic standards of testing. Ultimately, those who favored a change in course were outflanked (18).

A course similar to that which occurred with testing characterized the debate surrounding case reporting for HIV infection. Given the profound stigma that surrounded AIDS in the epidemic's first years, and the extent to which individuals with or at risk for HIV feared the social consequences of having their diagnoses made public, it is not surprising that confidentiality of AIDS-related information assumed great salience. From the pragmatic perspective of the public health officials it was crucial to preserve confidentiality as a way of ensuring that those at risk would come forward for testing and counseling (19). Those same concerns also had an effect on the ways in which ethicists viewed the matter. But from the perspective of the latter, protection of confidentiality was also a matter of fundamental principle. Privacy was a right of individuals that stemmed from the respect that was due to all persons.

But however central were the claims of privacy and the duty to protect confidentiality, they were not viewed as absolutes, even by ethicists. Conventionally accepted limits to those claims occurred when individuals with infectious diseases were reported by name to confidential public health registries. It was thus not surprising that despite concerns about privacy, little opposition existed in the epidemic's first years to making AIDS cases reportable by name (7). AIDS activists appreciated that such reporting was crucial to understanding the epidemiology of the new disease. The acceptance of AIDS case-reporting requirements was facilitated by the well-established record of state health departments in protecting such records from unwarranted disclosure.

With the inception of HIV testing, however, debate emerged about whether the names of all infected persons, regardless of whether they had received an AIDS diagnosis, should be reported. AIDS activists who accepted AIDS case reporting opposed HIV reporting because of heightened concerns about privacy, confidentiality, and discrimination. That was typically true as well of those who viewed the issue from the perspective of ethics. For them the potential public health benefits of reporting were too limited and the burden on those who would be the subject of reporting was too great to justify an abrogation of privacy.

While many public health officials, especially those who came from states with large AIDS caseloads, opposed HIV reporting because of its potential effect on the willingness of people to seek testing and counseling, some public health officials did become strong advocates of such reporting. Their claims sought to underscore the extent to which the public health benefits of HIV reporting would be like those that followed from more broadly conceived reporting requirements, such as those that applied to syphilis, tuberculosis, and AIDS itself (20).

As therapeutic advances began to emerge in the late 1980s, and as the logic of distinguishing between HIV and AIDS became increasingly difficult to sustain, fissures began to appear in the relatively broad and solid alliance against named HIV reporting. Thus, in 1989, New York City's Health Commissioner stated that the prospects of early clinical intervention warranted "a shift toward a disease-control approach to HIV infection along the lines of classic tuberculosis practices," including the "reporting of seropositives" (21). His proposal met with fierce and effective resistance in New York. Nevertheless, his perspective would increasingly be echoed at both the state and national levels.

At the end of November 1990, the CDC declared its support for HIV reporting, which it asserted could "enhance the ability of local, state and national agencies to project the level of required resources" for care and prevention services (22). Within a week, the House of Delegates of the American Medical Association endorsed the reporting of names as well, thus breaking with the traditional resistance of medical practitioners to such intrusions on the physician–patient relationship (23). In 1991, New Jersey became the first high-prevalence state to require HIV case reporting by name.

In the following years, the CDC continued to press for name-based reporting of HIV cases, supported by a growing number of public health officials. Indeed, the Council of State and Territorial Epidemiologists adopted resolutions in 1989, 1991, 1993, and 1995 encouraging states to consider the implementation of HIV reporting (24). Central to their argument was the assertion that AIDS case reporting captured an epidemic that was as much as a decade old and that an accurate picture of the incidence and prevalence of HIV infection—especially in light of the effect of treatment on the development of AIDS in those who were infected—required a surveillance system based on HIV case reporting. At the end of 1999, in the face of lingering opposition from most AIDS activists, the CDC finally proposed that all states put in place an HIV reporting system. And while it left open the possibility of reliance on unique identifiers that met strict performance criteria, it was clear that the use of names was viewed as preferable (25).

Nothing more tellingly underscores the change that had occurred and the extent to which the claims of public health necessity had trumped the arguments of privacy than an editorial jointly authored by a CDC official, an AIDS activist, and a lawyer-ethicist long involved in AIDS-related work that appeared in the *New England Journal of Medicine* in 1997:

We are at a defining moment of the epidemic of HIV infection and AIDS. With therapy that delays the progression to AIDS, mental illness, and death, HIV infection or AIDS is becoming a complex clinical disease that does not lend itself to monitoring based on end stage illness. Unless we revise our surveillance system, health authorities will not have reliable information about the prevalence of HIV infection. . . . To correct these deficiencies, we propose that all states require HIV case reporting. (26)

It was in confronting the issue of partner notification that those who came to AIDS from the perspective of bioethics found themselves endorsing positions that placed them at odds with those to whom they were more generally allied in shaping the exceptionalist strategy.

That respect for privacy and the protection of confidentiality were both pragmatically and ethically essential, was, as we have seen, a broadly held view in the epidemic's early years. What emerged as a source of contention in that period was the extent to which the protection of identifiable third parties who had been or were currently placed at risk for HIV by already infected individuals provided a warrant for public health interventions. This was not a new issue for ethicists; they had struggled with the question in the context of psychiatry in light of the so-called *Tarasoff* doctrine: that physicians who knew that their patients were about to inflict serious harm on other identifiable individuals had a duty to act to warn or protect (27). While opinions differed about the wisdom of such efforts, there was little principled objection to breaching confidentiality under such circumstances.

Thus in the mid to late 1980s, when many AIDS activists argued that the principle of confidentiality had to be inviolable, and when public health officials were loath to endorse legislative mandates *requiring* third-party notification, many ethicists suggested that protection of unsuspecting sexual partners took precedence over privacy: "When there are strong clinical grounds for believing that a specific contact has not been informed . . . the prudent course for the physician is to inform the contact of the positive serological status of the patient (28).

When, despite the opposition of most civil libertarians and activists, the American Medical Association's House of Delegates embraced the duty to warn in mid-1988, the association's president asserted,

This is a landmark in the history of medical ethics. We are saying for the first time that, because of the danger to the public health and the danger to unknowing partners who may be contaminated with this lethal disease, the physician may be required to violate patient confidentiality. The physician has a responsibility to inform the spouse. This is more than an option. This is a professional responsibility. (29)

Some states sought to meet the challenge of endangered third parties by enacting statutes that secured a "privilege to disclose." Under such laws physicians could, if they chose, breach confidentiality to warn unsuspecting individuals but would not be held liable if they failed to do so. So antagonistic were those committed to the primacy of privacy, to any breaches of confidentiality, that even such measures were viewed as anathema.

The depth of antagonism was further demonstrated by the deep suspicion of contact tracing programs, under which public health officials would notify those who had been placed at risk without divulging the identity of the individual who had imposed the risk. Such efforts were typically voluntary and relied on the willingness of the index patient to provide the name of his or her contacts.

Despite the four decades of experience with contact tracing, efforts to undertake such public health interventions in the context of AIDS met with fierce resistance in the first years of the epidemic. Opposition by gay leaders and civil liberties groups had a profound effect on the response of public health officials, especially in states with relatively large numbers of AIDS cases, where contact tracing efforts remained all but moribund (7). In part, the opposition was fueled by the fact that throughout most of the 1980s, no therapy could be offered to asymptomatic infected individuals. Thus, the role of contact tracing in the context of HIV infection differed radically from its role in the context of other STDs. In the latter case, effective treatments could be offered to notified partners. Once cured, such individuals would no longer pose a threat of transmission. In the case of HIV, nothing could be offered other than information about possible exposure to HIV.

For public health officials, who saw in such information an opportunity to target efforts to foster behavioral changes among individuals who were still engaging in high-risk behavior (behavior that could place both the individual contacted and future partners at risk) that was reason enough to undertake the process. For opponents of contact tracing, the very effort to reach out to such individuals represented a profound intrusion on privacy with little or no compensating benefit. The task of behavioral change, they asserted, could be achieved more effectively and efficiently through community-based HIV prevention efforts (30).

Early misapprehensions about the extent to which public health officials typically relied on overt coercion in the process of contact tracing, and the degree to which confidentiality might be compromised, had by the end of the 1980s all but vanished. With such concerns allayed, many gay leaders had come to recognize that partner notification, in fact, could be a "useful tool" in efforts to control AIDS (31).

By the late 1980s, the debate over contact tracing had shifted from one centered on the ethical issues of privacy to one focused on efficacy (32). That dispute was informed by questions that had already surfaced about the usefulness of contact tracing in the control of syphilis in populations where

individuals had large numbers of sexual partners, many of whom were anonymous (33).

In the issues of testing, reporting, and partner notification, those who were
drawn to AIDS from the field of bioethics were compelled, often for the first
time, to address matters involving public health. They were compelled to examine the limits of autonomy and privacy against the backdrop of an evolving epidemic, shifting epidemiological patterns, and clinical prospects. As the epidemic
affected increasing numbers of drug users and as the possibility of therapeutic
intervention improved, the exceptionalism of the first epidemic years began to
yield. Conventional public health practices were increasingly brought to bear, and
the relevance of ethics for the shaping of public policy on HIV and AIDS was
no longer so apparent to public health officials (23). Very different was the situation with respect to the conduct of research into HIV therapeutic interventions
and potential vaccines. Here the well-established interests and traditions of ethical analysis could be called on and would be viewed as having enduring importance. Strikingly, in the course of the encounter it would become clear that
matters considered settled would require reexamination.

The Ethics of Research

The ethical analysis of research involving human subjects emerged against a backdrop of torture, abuse, and scandal. From the Nuremberg Code, which sought to
set out the basic moral principles for research in the wake of the postwar trial of
Nazi doctors, to the establishment of the National Commission for the Protection of Human Subjects of Biomedical and Behavioral Research, created in the
wake of the 1973 revelation about the infamous Tuskegee syphilis experiment,
the need to protect potential subjects captured the attention of those appalled by
the practice of science. In 1978 it issued the *Belmont Report*, which codified a
set of ethical principles that sought to inform and guide the work of researchers
(34). Those principles provided the foundations for regulations subsequently enacted by the Department of Health and Human Services and the Food and Drug
Administration. At the core of those guidelines was the radical distinction between research designed to produce socially necessary, generalizable knowledge
and therapy designed to benefit individuals. Against the former, the *Belmont Report* held, individuals—especially those who were socially vulnerable—needed
protection against conscription. AIDS forced a reconsideration of this formulation.

The HIV epidemic provided the circumstances for the emergence of a broad
and potent political movement that sought to radically reshape the conditions under which research was undertaken. The role of the randomized clinical trial, the
importance of placebo controls, the centrality of academic research institutions,
the dominance of scientists over subjects, the sharp distinction between research

and therapy, and the protectionist ethos of the *Belmont Report* were all brought into question. Although scholars concerned with the methodological demands of sound research and ethicists committed to the protection of research subjects played a crucial role in the ensuing discussions, both as defenders of the received wisdom and as critics, the debate was largely driven by the articulate demands of those most threatened by AIDS (35). Most prominent were groups such as the People with AIDS Coalition and ACT UP, organizations made up primarily of white, gay men. They were joined by community-based physicians who identified closely with the plight of their patients.

What was so stunning—disconcerting to some, and exciting to others—was the rhythm of challenge and response. Rather than the careful exchange of academic arguments, there was the mobilization of disruptive and effective political protest. Most remarkable was the core demand. As Carol Levine noted, "The shortage of proven therapeutic alternatives for AIDS and the belief that trials are, in and of themselves, beneficial have led to the claim that people have a right to be research subjects. This is the exact opposite of the tradition started with Nuremberg—that people have a right *not* to be research subjects" (36). That striking reversal resulted in a rejection of the model of research conducted at remote academic centers, with restrictive (protective) standards of access, and strict adherence to the "gold standard" of the randomized clinical trial.

Blurring the distinction between research and treatment—expressed forcefully through the slogan "A Drug Trial Is Health Care Too"—those insistent on radical reform sought to open wide the points of entry to new "therapeutic" agents, both within and outside of clinical trials; they demanded that the paternalistic ethical warrant for the protection of the vulnerable from research be replaced by an ethical regime informed by respect for the autonomous choice of potential subjects who could weigh, for themselves, the potential risks and benefits of new treatments for HIV infection. Moreover, the revisionists demanded a basic reconceptualization of the relationship between researchers and subjects. In place of protocols imposed from above, they proposed a more egalitarian and democratic model in which negotiation would replace a scientific authority. Furthermore, the role of the carefully controlled clinical trial as providing protection against the widescale use of drugs whose safety and efficacy had not been proven no longer commanded unquestioned respect (37).

The new perspective did not go without challenge, of course. Some were concerned that the proposed regime would make the conduct of research so crucial to the needs of those with HIV/AIDS all but impossible (38); others feared that, in the absence of the now discredited (paternalistic) ethos, desperate individuals would be subject to deception (39).

But despite such resistance, the alliance of ethicists, activists, clinicians, and researchers who saw the need for change had seized the initiative. The reformist impulse was epitomized in an effort undertaken under the aegis of the American

Foundation for AIDS research, which sought to forge a new consensus on research ethics, one that would "entail a reappraisal of the ethical balance between
protecting the rights and welfare of subjects and expanding their options for pos-
sibly beneficial but still unproven drugs." When finally published in *IRB: A Review of Human Subjects Research* in 1991 (40), the report of the working group,
"Building a New Consensus: Ethical Principles and Policies for Clinical Research
on HIV/AIDS," reflected agreement on the need to replace the overly protective
and paternalistic ethos that had informed the regulation of research and to open
wide access to therapeutic trials to those who had previously been excluded or
who had faced severe restrictions: women, prisoners, drug users, and members
of racial and ethnic minority groups. Reflecting the political demands of AIDS
activists and an array of sympathetic researchers and clinicians, the consensus
not only stressed the critical importance of community consultation but argued
that such consultation should not be viewed as a way to obtain acceptance of an
already agreed-upon protocol; the task of shaping the protocol itself had to be a
"partnership."

The AIDS-inspired challenge to the ethics of research was not restricted to issues within the United States. With the globalization of the epidemic, it was inevitable that critical issues would emerge as research sponsored by wealthy nations took place in the world's poorest nations where the epidemic spread of HIV
took on alarming proportions. Would principles and practices developed in Western industrialized nations be applied to radically different settings? Would such
universalization represent a kind of ethical imperialism? How could the risks of
exploitation be precluded? These issues were sharply posed in the mid-1990s as
a number of, but by no means all, ethicists challenged international trials designed to determine whether a relatively simple and inexpensive AZT regimen—
much modified from that used in developed nations—could reduce the risks of
maternal–fetal transmission of HIV (41).

Because the trial involved the use of a placebo when an effective standard
of care had already been established, it was denounced as a reprehensible expression of the Tuskegee legacy. There is no question that a placebo-controlled
trial of efforts to reduce further vertical transmission in the wake of clinical
trial 076 would be considered unethical in the United States or another advanced industrial nation. No trial that denies access to the ACTG 076 regimen,
or to an intervention thought to hold the promise of being at least as effective
as, if not more effective than, the prevailing standard of care, would satisfy the
requirements of ethical review. The question posed was whether it is ethical to
conduct such a trial in a poor country where the ACTG 076 regimen is out of
reach as a potential therapy. Thus did Marcia Angell, the deputy editor of the
New England Journal of Medicine, assert, "Only when there is no known effective treatment is it ethical to compare a potential new treatment with a
placebo. When effective treatment exists, a placebo may not be used. Instead,

subjects in the control group of the study must receive the best known treatment" (42).

Angell and others who sided with her saw it as irrelevant that health care available in most third world countries provided nothing like health care available in industrialized countries. Citing the Declaration of Helsinki for authority, she noted that control groups had to be provided with the best current therapy, not simply that which is available locally. The shift in wording between "best" and "local" might appear to be slight, but the implications were profound. Acceptance of what she saw as "ethical relativism" could result in widespread exploitation of vulnerable third world populations for research programs that could not be carried out in the sponsor country:

All the rationalizations boil down to asserting that the end justifies the means—which it no more does in Africa than it did in Alabama. It is easy to see the findings of the Tuskegee study from a safe distance of 25 years. But those so offended by the comparison of the African research with Tuskegee have yet to show how these studies differ in their fundamental failure to protect the welfare of human subjects. (43)

The invective that characterized this controversy was striking, in part because, despite assertions to the contrary, this debate was not an instance of the ongoing clash between those who believed that a single Western-dominated ethical standard should apply to all research and others who held that ethical standards for research should reflect local values. Rather than a clash over basic principles, this was a dispute over the application of agreed-upon standards in radically different social conditions. Indeed, those ethicists who opposed Angell, many of whom had long advocated on behalf of vulnerable research subjects, asserted that the rigid reading of ethical principles corrupted the very purpose of such standards and would render all but impossible research that was critical for the most vulnerable.

Paralleling the debates over maternal–fetal transmission of HIV were those that surfaced over the ethics of AIDS vaccine trials. In this case, the focus was on those research participants who might become infected with HIV during a trial. On the one hand, there were those who argued that such individuals be provided with optimal care—the retroviral therapy available in the developed countries. On the other hand, there were those who asserted that care should reflect that which was consistent with what was available in the host nation (44). So divisive was this controversy that UNAIDS could not come to an agreement on the appropriate ethical norm and, indeed, had to settle for a procedural rather than a substantive solution, a solution that focused on how to reach acceptable agreement rather than one that put forth a standard to guide such deliberations (45).

Both the vaccine trial debate and the earlier controversy over maternal–fetal transmission inspired a vigorous discussion within the international ethics community over the standards that should govern the conduct of research involving rich sponsors and poor host nations, extending far beyond the AIDS epidemic. The World Medical Association engaged in an effort to rethink the Declaration of Helsinki. The Council of International Organizations of Medical Sciences (CIOMS) confronted the adequacy of its own earlier standards on such research. Finally, in the United States itself the National Bioethics Advisory Commission, established in 1995 by President Bill Clinton, devoted a special report to an unusually nuanced analysis of the moral complexity of international research in the global context characterized by vast inequalities in wealth and scientific infrastructure (46). Thus did AIDS serve as a catalytic force in the evolution of the ethics of human subjects research.

Access to Care

In the first years of the epidemic, there was little that medicine could offer those with HIV disease. That was the context, as we have noted, within which AIDS activists struggled to increase access to experimental trials. As the prospects for clinical intervention improved—first with the use of prophylactic treatment to prevent *Pneumocystis* pneumonia and other opportunistic infections and then with AZT, the first widely prescribed antiretroviral agent—it was inevitable that the inequities of the U.S. health-care system would be encountered.

The gross patterns of inequality in American health care had been the subject of analysis within bioethics since its emergence as a field in the 1970s. From the most egalitarian propositions (those that suggested that no health care should be available to any that was not available to all) to the least robust (which suggested a moral duty to ensure an "adequate" level of care to all without regard to the ability to pay), there was a basic consensus among bioethicists that prevailing conditions were unjust.

But unlike the impact of bioethics on the conduct of human subjects research, the ethical challenge to the U.S. health-care system had virtually no broad social or political resonance. Indeed, when the President's Commission for the Study of Ethical Problems in Medicine and Biomedical Research issued its report *Securing Access to Health Care* in 1983 (47), it went virtually unnoticed. And so tens of millions of Americans had no health insurance, and millions more were inadequately insured. Those who were poorly insured or uninsured had more difficulty in getting the care they needed, and they often did without.

This, then, was the context in which the medical needs of people with HIV disease had to be addressed. Some had private insurance, although they not infrequently faced efforts on the part of their insurers to deny them coverage for their HIV-related conditions; those who became impoverished because of their disease could qualify for Medicaid, but many remained unprotected (48). To meet their needs, special programs were developed, as described in Chapter 6. The federal government, through the Ryan White Care Act, directed hundreds of millions of dollars to localities to provide medical services. Among the initiatives under the act was the AIDS Drug Assistance Program (ADAP), which was designed to pay for AIDS-related medicines. But the patchwork effort was never adequate and left many without needed protection (49). Like the End Stage Renal Disease Program that ensured access to dialysis and transplantation regardless of the ability to pay, those programs left untouched the basic patterns of medical inequality.

When the protease inhibitors emerged in the mid-1990s and combination antiretroviral therapy became the standard of care, the system was strained to the limits. Medication costs alone for those receiving care could range from $10,000 to $15,000 a year (50). One review of dramatically improved therapeutic prospects added the caveat that the new achievements were important "at least for those socioeconomically privileged" (51). ADAP experienced persistent shortfalls in funding. When that was the case, it was necessary to resort to a host of rationing strategies. At one point, nearly half of the ADAP programs limited access to protease inhibitors (52). In 1996, the coordinator of Oregon's program explained that such coverage "would blow our budget out of the water" (53). A 1998 report by the National ADAP Monitoring Project found that fifteen states maintained waiting lists for entry to ADAP or for access to protease inhibitors. North Carolina, which had no formal waiting list, had simply stopped authorizing new clients for its ADAP. Only two state programs covered the fourteen drugs strongly recommended by the Public Health Service for the prevention of opportunistic infections (49).

As noted here, the remarkable advances in therapeutics have provided a critical element in the argument that the exceptionalism of the epidemic's early years is no longer appropriate. It is therefore a remarkable paradox that the very same achievements have set the stage for challenging the exceptionalist programs that—however inadequately—seek to ensure access to those same treatments. Thus in one analysis it was argued, "The absence of [benefits like those in the Ryan White Act] for persons with other stigmatizing diseases is troubling. We believe that this discrepancy leaves AIDS exceptionalism vulnerable to the accusation of injustice" (54). The "injustice" was underscored by Martin Delaney, founder of Project Inform, a community-based organization in San Francisco: "There are certainly other life-threatening diseases out there. Some of them kill a lot more people than AIDS does. So in one sense, it is almost an advantage to be HIV positive. It makes no sense" (55). These expressions of disquiet must be understood, at least in part, as a reflection of concern that in a changing political climate, where the American AIDS epidemic may no longer be seen as immediately threatening, unique services for those with HIV would become vulnerable unless they were embedded in a broader system of equitable health-care delivery. Indeed, when the Clinton administration rejected proposals to guarantee all people with HIV health insurance protection, it was asserted that such a move would raise "ethical" concerns given the prevailing inequities (56).

Just as the challenge of AIDS in the world's poorest nations compelled a confrontation with the prevailing ethical standards governing human subjects research, the global pandemic has provided the occasion for raising questions about global inequality in access to medical care. Of course, this maldistribution of medical care has long been recognized, and some ethical analysis has raised the question of the extent to which the principles of distributive justice could be used as a moral standard against which to judge such inequalities. But in an international context within which such claims were accorded little serious attention, where the political will to consider such matters was all but absent, ethical statements on access to health care seemed utterly quixotic. In a way that was unanticipated, AIDS, unlike the scourges of tuberculosis, malaria, and measles, appears to have altered that very context.

The availability of powerful and effective antiretroviral therapies in the richest nations where the HIV epidemic was smaller and their inaccessibility, because of cost and infrastructural requirements, in the poorest nations where the burden of HIV was greatest, set the stage for the emergence of an international activist movement demanding the end to such inequality, the slashing of AIDS drug prices, and the creation of a vast global fund to make anti-HIV drugs available to the world's poorest. Involved were not only challenges to the global pharmaceutical industry, the World Trade Organization, and the international treaty governing patent rights, but to the world's powerful industrial nations. The most remarkable expressions of the impact of these challenges was the agreement reached by the World Health Organization and the World Trade Organization on differential drug pricing in 2001 (57) and the concomitant effort on the part of the Secretary General of the United Nations to amass a "global fund" of $7 to $10 billion a year to meet the challenge of AIDS, malaria, and tuberculosis (58).

Whether such efforts will prove fruitful cannot, at this juncture, be known. But it is clear that the dimensions of the tragedy of AIDS in Africa; the willingness of activists in many nations to link arms in a common struggle; and the example of Brazil, which has challenged the prerogatives of the pharmaceutical industry and which has provided antiretroviral therapies to all of its infected citizens, have served to create a sociopolitical context within which the most basic concepts of international equity can be taken seriously. In so doing, the campaign for access to AIDS drugs has given political heft to ethical discussion of justice beyond borders.

Conclusions

Since the first reports of what would become known as AIDS appeared in *Morbidity and Mortality Weekly Report*, many of those who worked in the field of bioethics were compelled to confront issues posed by the epidemic. That they affected the shaping of policy is amply demonstrated in this chapter. How lasting that effect will be is far less certain. But what has been the impact of the epidemic on the world of ethics generally, and of public health ethics more specifically?

In an important way, the epidemic years have provided an object lesson on the importance of social context for ethical analysis—on the poverty of analysis that is uninformed by such understanding. No effort to appreciate the ethical challenges posed by AIDS could have been adequate had the unique needs and fears of those most at risk not been taken into account. No consideration of the claims of privacy and its limits could have been complete had the unique history of gay men not been attended to. Nor would an ethical analysis that had ignored the vulnerable status of women, especially poor minority women, been sufficient to the task at hand.

The AIDS epidemic taught an important lesson to ethicists about the necessity of engaging those most at risk in ongoing discussion. Such discussion served the ends of good analysis by providing insights that might not otherwise have been available. More important, the needs and claims of those most at risk could often set the agenda for ethical discussion. That was certainly the case with regard to clinical research. In a fundamental sense, then, AIDS provided insight into the virtues and limits of democratic discourse.

Perhaps the greatest impact of AIDS on ethics, however, may in the long run be found in the way it has inspired a serious discussion of the ethics of public health as distinct from an ethics of the clinical relationship. To be sure, there were discussions of the ethics of public health before AIDS—analyses spurred by motorcycle helmet and seat belt laws and by occupational health regulation, for example. But while legions were drawn to clinical issues, those who thought of ethical issues bearing on public health, however episodically, could be counted on one's hands. That discussion is still at a very formative stage, and it remains unclear what direction it will take. For example, it is difficult to discern whether a common set of principles will animate the field in the way that was true for bioethics, although it is clear that whatever conceptual frame emerges will require something beyond the individualism that served to inform the field of clinical ethics.

Here it is worth noting that among the most notable developments since the epidemic took hold has been the effort to demonstrate the linkage between human rights and public health. The precise nature of that relationship, which underscores the importance of both classical political rights and social equality for public health, is beyond the scope of this chapter. But what must be emphasized is the fact that it was in the confrontation with the AIDS epidemic that this challenging outlook took form.

Whatever substantive principles come to inform the ethics of public health, it is the very recognition that the ethics of public health warrant careful and ongoing discussion that represents a development of singular significance. To appreciate the role of values in the shaping of public policies designed to advance communal health, to understand that such values are commonly in tension, will set the stage for the kind of effort that had such a profound effect on medicine and clinical research.

Bioethics was borne of human suffering and tragedy. So, too, does it appear that will be the case for public health ethics. These precious achievements underscore the human capacity to wrest some good from the misery imposed by nature and artifice.

References

1. Rothman DJ: *Strangers at the Bedside.* Basic Books, New York, 1991.
2. Jonsen AR: *The Birth of Bioethics.* Oxford University Press, New York, 1998.
3. Karst KL: The freedom of intimate association. *Yale Law Rev* 89: 624–692, 1980.
4. Cited in Merritt DJ: The constitutional balance between health and liberty. *Hastings Cent Rep* 16: S2–10, 1986.
5. Merritt DJ: Communicable disease and constitutional law: controlling AIDS. *New York Univ Law Rev* 61: 739–799, 1986.
6. Bayer R: Public health policy and the AIDS epidemic: an end to HIV exceptionalism? *N Engl J Med* 324: 1500–1504, 1991.
7. Bayer R: *Private Acts, Social Consequences: AIDS and the Politics of Public Health.* Rutgers University Press, New Brunswick, NJ, 1989, pp. 101–136.
8. Bayer R, Levine C, and Wolf S: HIV antibody screening: an ethical framework for evaluating proposed programs. *JAMA* 256: 1768–1774, 1986.
9. Faden RR, Kass NE, Acuff KL, et al.: HIV Infection and childbearing: a proposal for public policy and clinical practice. In Faden RR and Kass NE (eds.): *HIV, AIDS and Childbearing: Public Policy, Private Lives.* Oxford University Press, New York, 1996, pp. 447–461.
10. Centers for Disease Control and Prevention: Additional recommendations to reduce sexual and drug abuse-related transmission of human T-lymphotropic virus type III/lymphadenopathy associated virus. *Morb Mortal Wkly Rep* 35: 152–155, 1986.
11. Bayer R: Women's rights, babies' interests: ethics, politics, and science in the debate of newborn HIV screening. In Minkoff HL, DeHovitz JA, and Duerr A (eds.): *HIV Infection in Women.* Raven Press, New York, 1995, pp. 293–307.
12. Hegearty M and Abrams E: Caring for HIV-infected women and children. *N Engl J Med* 326: 887–888, 1992.
13. New York Governor's Program, Bill No 123, 1996.
14. Centers for Disease Control: Zidovudine for the prevention of HIV transmission from mother to infant. *Morb Mortal Wkly Rep* 43: 285–287, 1994.
15. Minkoff H and Willoughby A: Pediatric HIV disease, zidovudine in pregnancy, and unblinding heelstick surveys: reframing the debate on prenatal HIV testing. *JAMA* 274: 1165–1168, 1995.
16. Shelton DL: Delegates push mandatory HIV testing for pregnant women: American Medical Association House of Delegates vote: annual meeting news. *Am Med News* 31: 1, 1996.
17. Institute of Medicine: *Reducing the Odds: Preventing Perinatal Transmission of HIV in the United States.* National Academy Press, Washington DC, 1998.

18. Centers for Disease Control and Prevention: Revised guidelines for HIV counseling, testing, and referral. *Morb Mortal Wkly Rep* 50: 1–58, 2001

19. Institute of Medicine: *Confronting AIDS.* National Academy Press, Washington DC, 1986.

20. Vernon T: Remarks. In Hummell R, Leavy W, Rampola R, and Chorost S (eds.): *AIDS: Impact on Public Policy.* Plenum Press, New York, 1986.

21. Joseph SC: Remarks presented at the Fifth International Conference on AIDS, Montreal, Quebec, June 4–9, 1989.

22. Centers for Disease Control and Prevention: Update: public health surveillance for HIV infection: United States, 1989 and 1990. *Morb Mortal Wkly Rep* 39: 853–861, 1990.

23. Bayer R: Clinical progress and the future of HIV exceptionalism. *Arch Intern Med* 159: 1042–1048, 1999.

24. Council of State and Territorial Epidemiologists, unpublished data, 1997.

25. Centers for Disease Control and Prevention: Guidelines for national human immunodeficiency virus case surveillance, including monitoring for Human Immunodeficiency Virus infection and Acquired Immune Deficiency Syndrome. *Morb Mortal Wkly Rep* 48: 1–28, 1999.

26. Gostin LO, Wrad JW, and Baker AC: National HIV case reporting for the United States: a defining moment in the history of the epidemic. *N Engl J Med* 337: 1162–1167, 1997.

27. *Tarasoff v. Regents of California*, 188 Cal Rptr 129 (Cal Sup Ct 1974).

28. Gostin L and Curran W: AIDS screening, confidentiality and the duty to warn. *Am J Pub Health* 77: 361–365, 1987.

29. *New York Times*, July 1, 1988, p. A1.

30. Bayer R and Toomey KE: HIV prevention and the two faces of partner notification. *Am J Pub Health* 82: 1158–1164, 1992.

31. Schram N: Partner notification can be useful tool against AIDS spread. *Los Angeles Times*, June 28, 1988, p. 7.

32. *Contact Tracing and Partner Notification.* American Public Health Association, Washington DC, 1988.

33. Andrus JK, Fleming DW, Harger DR et al.: Partner notification: can it control syphilis? *Ann Intern Med* 112: 539–543, 1990.

34. National Commission for the Protection of Human Subjects: *The Belmont Report: Ethical Principles and Guidelines for the Protection of Human Subjects.* U.S. Government Printing Office, Washington, DC, 1979.

35. Epstein S: *Impure Science: AIDS, Activism, and the Politics of Knowledge.* University of California Press, Berkeley, 1996.

36. Levine C: Has AIDS changed the ethics of human subjects research? *Law, Med Health Care* 16: 167–173, 1988.

37. Bayer R: Beyond the burdens of protection: AIDS and the ethics of research. *Eval Rev* 14: 443–446, 1990.

38. Parallel track system defended. *CDC AIDS Wkly*, December 11, 1989.

39. Annas GJ: Faith (healing), hope and charity at the FDA: the politics of AIDS drug trials. *Villanova Law Rev* 34: 771–797, 1989.

40. Levine C, Dubler NN, and Levine RJ: Building a new consensus: ethical principles and policies for clinical research on HIV/AIDS. *IRB* 13: 1–17, 1991.

41. Bayer R: The debate over maternal–fetal HIV transmission prevention trials in Africa, Asia and the Caribbean: racist exploitation or exploitation of racism? *Am J Pub Health* 88: 567–570, 1998.

42. Angell M: The ethics of clinical research in the third world. *N Engl J Med* 337: 847–849, 1997.

43. Angell M: Tuskegee revisited. *Wall Street Journal*, October 28, 1997, p. A22.

44. Bayer R: Ethical challenges of HIV vaccine trials in less developed nations: conflict and consensus in the international arena. *AIDS* 14: 1051–1057, 2000.

45. UNAIDS: *Ethical Considerations in HIV Preventive Vaccine Research*, 2000.

46. National Bioethics Advisory Commission: *Ethical and Policy Issues in International Research: Clinical Trials in Developing Countries.* Bethesda, MD, 2001.

47. President's Commission for the Study of Ethical Problems in Medicine and Biomedical Research: *Securing Access to Health Care*, 1983.

48. Green J and Arno PS: The "medicaidization" of AIDS: trends in the financing of HIV-related medical care. *JAMA* 264: 1261–1266, 1990.

49. National ADAP Monitoring Project: *Interim Technical Report.* Kaiser Family Foundation, Menlo Park, CA, 1998.

50. Deeks SG, Smith M, Holodny M, and Kahn JO: HIV-1 protease inhibitors: a review for clinicians. *JAMA* 277: 145–153, 1997.

51. Richman DD: HIV therapeutics. *Science* 272: 1886–1888, 1996.

52. Carton B: New AIDS drugs bring hope to Provincetown, but unexpected woes. *Wall Street Journal*, October 3, 1996, p. A1.

53. Goldstein A: New treatments put AIDS program in a dilemma. *Washington Post*, August 15, 1996, p. A1.

54. Casarett DJ and Lantos JD: Have we treated AIDS too well? Rationing and the future of AIDS exceptionalism. *Ann Intern Med* 128: 756–759, 1998.

55. Stolberg SG: White House drops plan for Medicaid to cover cost of AIDS drugs for poor. *New York Times*, December 6, 1997, p. 14.

56. Birmingham K: Clinton's spending on AIDS care goes awry. *Nat Med* 4: 138, 1998.

57. World Health Organization and World Trade Organization Secretariats: *Report of the Workshop on Differential Pricing and Financing of Essential Drugs.* Hosbjor, Norway, 2001.

58. The United Nations Secretary General to lead the fight against HIV/AIDS. *UNAIDS Press Release*, April 5, 2001.

8

Contributions of HIV Prevention Evaluation to Public Health Program Evaluation

LAURA C. LEVITON AND MARY E. GUINAN

In this chapter we describe the evaluation of HIV prevention efforts and suggest ways in which it has contributed to evaluation in public health generally. Although important questions about evaluation also arise in the context of HIV treatment and care programs, they will not be the focus of this chapter. In the first section we describe the context of the contributions. In the middle section, we appraise the contributions made by research demonstrations and their evaluation in HIV prevention. In the final section, we discuss the shift over time to established, large-scale programs for HIV prevention and describe how the increase in program dollars has led to increased evaluation capacity at national, regional, state and local levels.

The Contributions of HIV Prevention Evaluation

Evaluation of HIV prevention efforts ("HIV prevention evaluation") has contributed to evaluation of public health programs ("public health evaluation") in several ways. Despite chronic methodological problems, HIV prevention evaluation has helped expand the array of program evaluation methods. In addition, evaluation evidence from research projects in HIV prevention has helped to reduce uncertainty about the value of key public health practices. In research projects, HIV prevention evaluation has helped to explicate program theory, as well as behavioral theories applied to public health. In the context of large-scale programs, HIV prevention evaluation has helped to guide practitioners in the choice of effective (evaluated) program models. It has increased public health evaluation capacity at all levels. Finally, HIV prevention evaluation has pointed to some new opportunities and superior models for public health evaluation that may not be widely appreciated.

HIV prevention evaluation contributed to changes in public health evaluation, but that does not imply that it was the single cause for such changes. Evaluation is embedded in the context of program, policy, and practice, and it rarely contributes to knowledge independent of the context (1–3). Evaluation makes incremental changes in knowledge, methods, and the shaping of programs. Also, many of these contributions are invisible to those who are not directly involved in their development. HIV prevention evaluation developed side by side with evaluation of other public health programs, resulting in an interchange of methods and practice-based knowledge. Such interchanges between areas are often invisible because researchers dealing with one prevention problem tend not to cite researchers in other areas, and because government agencies primarily cite their own products (1,3).

However, we can trace the influence of HIV prevention evaluations using specific milestone events and seminal documents. Within the United States, for example, HIV researchers contributed significantly to evaluation in public health by soliciting the best available thinking from practicing evaluation methodologists. From the outset, the Institute of Medicine (4) and the National Center for Health Services Research (5) gave seminal guidance. HIV researchers solicited expertise on measurement that greatly increased the usefulness and precision of their work (6–8). Most recently, a working group of the Centers for Disease Control and Prevention (CDC) developed a widely disseminated consensus on the state of the art in public health evaluation, with authorship by several researchers who had done extensive evaluation of HIV prevention methods (9).

Like evaluation in most policy sectors, evaluation as it developed in the field of HIV prevention is best described as "a mixed bag" (1,10). Evaluation has always come at the cost of numerous false starts, poor practice, and then a growing recognition of how the process might be improved. One can point to many methodological flaws in HIV prevention evaluation, some of which could have been avoided by a more careful reading of the evaluation literature. However, those false starts are not the focus of this chapter. In spite of these problems, HIV has indeed been influential because it forced evaluation issues onto the center stage of public health. HIV prevention catalyzed public health evaluation because of the intense scrutiny it received, the very large new investments in programming, the consequent demands by policymakers to seek evidence of effectiveness, the urgency and variety of evaluation questions, and the large number and diversity of the organizations involved in HIV prevention.

The United States dominates the field of evaluation, so it should come as no surprise that it also dominates evaluation of HIV prevention (11). However, advances in evaluation are by no means "all-American." European social scientists, for example, were far in advance of Americans in exploring the epistemology of evaluation (12). As seen in the final section of this chapter, their contributions helped answer essential challenges posed by evaluating HIV prevention and other public health programs in many cultures, by the need for participatory evaluation, and by the efforts to increase evaluation capacity closer to the "street level" of service provision.

Internationally, the countries with the most developed public health infrastructure tend to undertake the most public health evaluation (11). This is not to dismiss the deficits in HIV prevention infrastructure, even in wealthy countries. Moreover, we will discuss how the poorest nations have sometimes provided the best insights on HIV prevention programs and their evaluation. Before the AIDS epidemic, these included important outreach strategies and new qualitative methods. And since then, the lack of resources has sometimes forced ambitious innovations in HIV prevention and rigorous tests of effectiveness. These can be seen, for example, in the areas of HIV testing and counseling, treatment of sexually transmitted diseases to prevent HIV, and behavioral interventions (13–15).

Evaluation Definition and Approaches

Jargon and arbitrary distinctions abound in evaluation, so there is a need to define what we are talking about. The most common definition of evaluation is the systematic assessment of the value of an object or activity (16), and it is most commonly applied to organized efforts to address a need or problem, such as HIV transmission (17). The organized effort can be a practice, program element, component, or activity, such as outreach to people at risk of HIV in order to provide intervention (18); a pilot project, feasibility study, or research demonstration such as the AIDS Community Demonstration Projects conducted by the CDC (19); an established program aimed at serving entire populations, such as the brothel-based "100 percent condom" program of Thailand (14); or a policy, such as European countries' endorsement of needle exchange programs (20), or a school system's policy permitting health curricula to mention the effectiveness of condoms in preventing HIV infection (21).

Evaluations of these efforts take place at local, state, national, and international levels. They can focus on inputs, (such as the resources being applied to the problem); implementation of HIV prevention activities (often termed process); a variety of outcomes (impacts, outputs), for which the terminology differs often in contradictory fashion across fields; and cost-utility analysis, including the measurement of program costs, cost-benefit, and cost-effectiveness. This last area, which is critically important to the agencies that fund HIV prevention, blends into policy analysis (17,22). A variety of methods and approaches are commonly employed in evaluation, and all of these have been useful in HIV prevention. They include randomized field experiments and quasi-experimental designs (23–25); systematic planning for evaluation and comprehensive evaluation (17,26,27); issues of external validity and replication of models in new locations (28); and case study and qualitative approaches (29,30), participatory approaches (31), and approaches to deal with the organizational, political, and human constraints on production of useful evaluation (1,32,33).

Evaluations of HIV Prevention Research Demonstrations

Program Theory: A Critical Contribution to Public Health Evaluation

It is our belief that HIV prevention stimulated the increased use of program theory in public health evaluation. A program theory is a set of statements about *(a)* forces that affect the problem the program hopes to change; *(b)* program activities that are presumed to affect those forces; and *(c)* logical linkages between program activities, changes in those forces and changes in the overall problem. The very first comprehensive monograph on program evaluation introduced the idea of program theory in 1967, and it is worth recalling that it was written by a public health sociologist (34). However, the explicit use of program theory in public health evaluation was not common until the mid-1990s. From the beginning of HIV/AIDS, policy-makers had urgently demanded a base of evidence for the viability of HIV prevention programs, and program theory was viewed as a central feature of the evidence base. These demands drove the use of program theory for prevention more generally (35). In present-day HIV prevention, program theory and the related concept of logic models are often the primary bases for determining a useful evaluation focus, and it is our impression that they have been more prevalent in HIV prevention than in other areas of public health. Furthermore, program theory, after it has been subjected to evaluation, has been key to the refinement and targeting of HIV prevention in the United States and to some degree, internationally.

Increased use of program theory was a key development for public health evaluation because program theory is intimately tied to high-quality evaluation. Program theory and logic models explicitly describe assumptions about the underlying problem, then relate program inputs and implementation to immediate, intermediate, and ultimate outcomes. Focusing on the theory underlying a program has been highly useful for program development and evaluation planning (26,27,36), for enhancing our ability to generalize and adapt models to new populations and settings (28), for improved quantitative analysis (37,38), and as more useful qualitative analysis (33).

Contributions to the Evaluation of Public Health Practice

Evaluation in public health originated in the nineteenth century with the need for statistical indicators of community health (34). Early in the twentieth century, public health evaluation focused primarily on monitoring the degree to which public health workers adhered to standards (34). This continues as a concern into the twenty-first century, especially in areas such as HIV counseling and testing programs (13,39). Although some process and outcome evaluations of public health programs were conducted in the United States in the 1950s, the U.S. "Great Society" programs of the 1960s focused attention squarely on the question of outcomes (1,34). Public health program evaluations in this era foreshadowed some of the evaluation challenges that would later be seen in the HIV epidemic. The public health practices that were the focus of these evaluations were largely eclipsed in the early 1980s, but because of HIV they reemerged with new urgency, more widespread attention, and new evaluation methodology. Two important evaluation topics in particular have revived and extended public health practice: community participation and increased access through outreach strategies.

Assessing the inclusiveness and quality of community participation in urban health service systems was a key focus for evaluation of several Great Society health programs (40,41). Given the World Health Organization's emphasis on community participation, it should come as no surprise that international health also developed models to evaluate community participation (42,43). In the HIV epidemic, almost from the beginning, policy-makers understood how important it was to involve the affected communities to gain their buy-in and support. The results of research demonstrations certainly supported this assumption (19). Today an important evaluation focus concerns the participation of communities affected by the HIV epidemic, a key requirement of CDC's Community Planning Process (see Chapter 3). In the United States, other health promotion programs now focus on evaluating community participation to a modest degree, but not uniformly and seldom to meet a requirement (44,45). Leaders in public health practice in the United States are attempting to incorporate methods of citizen participation and its evaluation on a voluntary basis (46–50); however, CDC's requirement of community participation in planning HIV prevention programs has forced evaluation of this indicator on a broader scale by many more grantees and contractors (51,52).

A program and evaluation theme of the Great Society concerned access to health care (53,54). One strategy to increase access was employment of indigenous paraprofessionals, and evaluation established their effectiveness in several health-care and prevention roles (55–57). Outreach workers and lay health educators have never disappeared entirely from the scene: their role has been evaluated in U.S. maternal and child health (58), and they have a prominent role in developing nations (59).

In coping with HIV transmission, public health practitioners' mindset about access had to change, because the populations at risk were unlikely to present themselves to formal organizations. HIV prevention programs therefore employed a variety of outreach techniques, as seen in studies of gay and bisexual men (4,60), injection drug users (IDUs) (61–63), and women at risk (64), and in people being treated for STD around the globe (14). Outreach has become a more important focus for public health evaluation generally (18). In addition, key evaluation findings derived from outreach in HIV prevention: first, that employing members or former members of the populations at risk is important (19,61–63); second, that volunteer outreach workers could often extend the influence of social marketing and health education (19,65); and third, that lay health educators with professional backup could follow a complex protocol for HIV prevention with excellent fidelity (66).

Evaluation of HIV prevention, at least in the United States, shares another significant feature with the Great Society programs: they have undergone scrutiny that is arguably out of proportion to actual expenditures. All too often, it is the new, the innovative, and the less politically entrenched programs that are subjected to evaluation because they are most frequently held accountable for results and must justify the allocation of resources (1). In the case of the Great Society, it was merely that the programs challenged the status quo; HIV prevention, however, posed hotly debated questions about morality. Although HIV prevention budget lines have gained at least some financial and political stability, many questions persist about the evidence for and successful adaptation of HIV prevention. These questions have stimulated an urgency to develop methods that cost less and represent less response burden from recipient agencies than do the more prevalent evaluation methods (67,68).

Health Behavior and Health Promotion Interventions before and after HIV

HIV prevention and its evaluation contributed to the growth of behavioral applications in public health. Behavioral scientists began to apply theories and methods to chronic disease in the 1970s, but they had little effect on public health until the establishment of the U.S. Office of Health Promotion and Disease Prevention in the late 1970s, and the publication in 1980 of the PRECEDE model for health promotion planning. PRECEDE ("Predisposing, Reinforcing and Enabling Constructs in Ecosystem Diagnosis and Evaluation") is a framework that forces planners to consider the behavioral factors contributing to a health problem, analyze the specific forces maintaining the behavioral factors, and select for intervention those forces that are both important and modifiable. PRECEDE made behavioral science accessible to public health at large and married behavioral theory to public health application (69). Yet for several reasons, behavior and lifestyle changes as primary outcomes for evaluation still did not gain widespread currency in public health until the HIV epidemic. First, prevention of chronic disease was not a primary focus for most public health agencies. Second, most public health practice had no theory of behavior change beyond simple exhortation and a medical model of treatment (70,71). Third, many researchers in medicine and public health did not view behavioral change as "hard data" because it was so often self-reported and open to challenge. Yet, as publications repeat over and over, interventions to promote behavior change continue to be the major HIV prevention approaches available on a wide scale, and behavioral outcomes are the most feasible to evaluate in most situations (4).

Dating from its initial HIV prevention research projects funded in 1985, the CDC began widespread use of behavioral outcomes for evaluation of its publicly funded HIV prevention programs. Several key events demonstrate how the HIV epidemic increased the sense of urgency to apply behavioral theory to health behaviors and to develop relevant outcome measures. In 1988 the CDC invited several prominent behavioral theorists to identify the common elements of their theories that could be applied in HIV prevention interventions across populations and settings (72). These were incorporated into an applied program theory for HIV prevention and were used to design the AIDS Community Demonstration Projects, as well as later projects (19,65,66). In 1991, a meeting of behavioral theorists at the National Institute of Mental Health developed a similar but more elaborated framework (73). These frameworks were the first to integrate the predominant behavioral theories to address an applied behavioral problem, so their contribution far outstrips even public health applications. They have greatly improved program theory for health promotion programs and have provided at least some consensus on evaluation outcomes.

The application of behavioral theory in HIV prevention probably helped to increase the visibility of its application to chronic disease within the wider public health field. A milestone came in 1998, when chronic disease specialists initiated CDC's first large scientific conference on behavioral science applications to pubic health. Cosponsored by the major behavioral science professional associations, with high visibility and attendance by a broad array of public health professionals, the meeting signaled public health's increased acceptance of behavioral science and its research methods (74).

Some Key Contributions of HIV Prevention to Evaluation of Health Promotion

Technically, the evaluation of behavior change in HIV prevention efforts has often been very unsatisfactory. The supposed difficulties of evaluation in real-world settings do not excuse the continuing problem of validating self-report, the lack of consensus on measurement of behaviors, or the fact that studies still continue to incorporate questionable designs and analyses that give misleading conclusions when superior methods are available (23–25,75,76). In spite of these problems, evaluation in HIV prevention has also contributed important advances: in the use of qualitative methods, in appropriate sampling, and in determining the scale and intensity of interventions to reach entire populations or communities.

In general, qualitative methods for both planning and evaluating HIV prevention became far advanced and useful, in comparison to those employed in chronic disease prevention. Formal ethnographic methods (as anthropologists usually employ them) are lengthy and cumbersome for the planning and evaluation needs of an epidemic on the move (77). As such, rapid qualitative techniques were developed to meet the needs of HIV prevention evaluation (78,79), some of which derived from international public health programs for nutrition and primary health care (80). Qualitative techniques tend to be more flexible than quantitative data collection protocols and are especially important at the formative stage of HIV prevention program evaluation.

Because of improved qualitative methods, HIV researchers learned where individuals at risk would congregate on given days and times. In this way, qualitative advances permitted an important advance in quantitative methods, including probability sampling and, specifically, cluster sampling to evaluate behavior changes in difficult-to-reach populations (62,81). Studies of behavior often focus on convenience samples, employing motivated volunteers or snowball samples (81). Early in the investigation of interventions on health risks, such samples can be justified because the focus is on internal validity (Does intervention cause risk reduction?), not external validity (To what populations can findings be generalized?) (28,82). However, public health aims to understand the prevalence of changes in populations, and this is an external validity question (70).

Most studies in behavioral medicine were intensive individual applications, raising the evaluative question of whether they could be applied to entire populations at a reasonable cost (70). To reach entire populations, chronic disease prevention researchers employed social marketing and comprehensive community-based approaches (83). However, the resultant changes in awareness, behavior, and health status were often disappointing. Since entire cities and states were targeted and assessed, interventions may not have reached the entire population that was sampled for study, or they may not have reached the population with sufficient intensity and duration to matter (84).

Some studies of social marketing and community-based HIV prevention appear to have greater intervention effects than those seen in chronic disease prevention (15,19,60,65). In contrast to social marketing in chronic disease prevention, entire populations are rarely the units of intervention, assignment, and analysis for HIV risk reduction. The behavior of entire populations does not put people at risk of HIV (with the possible exception of high-prevalence countries). Instead, HIV intervention often targets specific social networks or neighborhoods where infection and high-risk behaviors are most prevalent. Intervention at this level may be more realistic in its intensity and duration than larger-scale interventions. To evaluate population changes, individual level assessment is too small, and city and state level assessment is too big; but perhaps community and network level assessments are "just right."

Private, Hidden, and Illegal Behaviors: Analysis and Intervention

Improvements in the study and measurement of sexual behavior were directly motivated by the emergency of HIV (85). Dating from the onset of AIDS, one sees improvements in valid measurement of sexual behavior and appropriate sampling of respondents (86), as well as ethnographic studies of gender relations across cultures (87). Some important research on intimate relationships and sexual attraction did predate the epidemic (88). However, both HIV epidemiology and research demonstrations cast light on the measurement of risk within intimate relationships, as well as cultural and national variations in sexual mixing and power relationships (15). These insights have general importance for reproductive health and for women's health and well-being.

   HIV prevention research projects also helped launch an important body of research on substance abuse treatment effectiveness. Before AIDS, a few large outcome studies had concluded that people who receive substance abuse treatment tend to do better than those who do not, that in-patient and outpatient treatments are about equally effective, and that those who stay in treatment longer do better (89). However, very little was known about how treatment interacts with individual characteristics; for example, is the effect of longer treatment a real treatment effect, or is it self-selection by users who are more motivated to stick with treatment? These issues have great importance for resource allocation and reimbursement of services.

   In the late 1980s and early 1990s, the National Institute on Drug Abuse funded a large number of demonstration projects to teach drug users outside treatment how to avoid HIV infection (61). A large proportion of these drug users reported previous treatment experiences, casting light on the potential selection artifacts in the previous outcome studies (63). This finding also drove home the conclusion that most people need to try several times to quit using drugs. Along with other information, these studies provided the justification to initiate a clinical trials network for more rigorous testing and better client follow up (90–92).

Summary of Contributions

In the application of program theory and behavioral theory to public health evaluation, the urgency and visibility of HIV prevention probably increased the speed of improvements that were already under way. Evaluation of HIV prevention research projects contributed in a different way by decreasing uncertainty about effective public health practices. Yet a third kind of contribution was to improve our understanding of sexual behavior and drug treatment. Finally, the improve-

ments in methodology that resulted from HIV prevention research demonstrations are applicable to the rest of public health.

Evaluation in Established HIV Prevention Programs

Shifting from Research Projects to Established Programs

HIV prevention evaluation has developed in ways similar to evaluation in other
policy sectors. When a problem is fairly new and solutions are poorly understood,
research projects and pilot studies are common (17). As knowledge accrues about
how to address the problem, national and international programs emerge, funded
by governments and international donors and implemented by a wide variety of
organizations and practitioners, the "street level" of implementation. As large-
scale programs emerge, evaluation needs often shift, because funders and policy-
makers encounter the need to ensure that implementation proceeds as they intended (1,10,17,26,27). Even in the most centralized service systems, funders
usually lack direct control over "street level" implementation, and there may be
a variety of barriers to implementation. The need arises for monitoring to ensure
high-quality implementation and progress on outcomes (17), often by requiring
the funded organizations to submit evaluation reports. The need also arises to
provide guidance to the "street level" about how to improve program implementation. In combination, these challenges tend to increase the need for evaluation capacity, not only within the funding organizations but also in the funded
organizations that are closer to the "street level" of implementation.

In HIV prevention, this shift in emphasis has produced important contributions
to public health evaluation generally. Over time, the CDC, the World Bank, the
World Health Organization, and other donors have distributed substantial money
for prevention (see Chapter 1). To reach entire populations with intervention,
funds often need to go to regional and local organizations, which are typically
closer to the problem, are trusted by the population, and may have special expertise to engage people on HIV prevention. Yet, implementation is outside the
direct control of national and state governments and funding agencies, which are
faced with the need to ensure that the money was spent well.

The shift in evaluation tasks has produced at least four specific contributions
to public health evaluation: (1) using the evidence base to guide allocation of resources, (2) guiding grantees to the evidence-based prevention models, (3) evaluating the external validity of evidence-based models, and (4) creating new evaluation capacity at all levels, most notably at the state and local level, closer to
"street level" implementation of prevention. While it is true that other public
health programs are also helping to build evaluation capacity, the influence of
HIV is noteworthy because of the scope of resources and the scale of evaluations
required by the donor organizations.

Evidence-Based Resource Allocation

Nationally and internationally, funders of HIV prevention have used the evidence base concerning effectiveness to argue for resources, to allocate those resources rationally, and to encourage the funded organizations to adopt evidence-based prevention models. To achieve these ends, they identify "best practices," undertake literature reviews, and commission meta-analyses to identify interventions with documented success at preventing HIV (see Chapter 4). These reviews keep growing as new evidence is added (93).

The need to allocate resources more rationally and to argue from the evidence for additional resources is leading to new developments and more widespread applications of cost-utility analysis in public health evaluation (22,94,95). Within the HIV arena, policy-makers were asking why new cases continued to arise when so much money was being allocated and when hard decisions needed to be made about the most effective ways to spend the money. HIV researchers contributed to important CDC guidance on cost utility (35). Before HIV, important work on cost utility was already developed in chronic disease prevention (96,97). However, cost-utility evaluations and the tools to make them possible were not commonly employed in public health programs. HIV helped stimulate an overall concern for resource allocation in public health, and HIV researchers helped persuade and lead practitioners to use the CDC guidance on cost utility.

From Evidence Base to Application: Use of Evaluation Findings

The premise of the cost-utility models is that local service providers, including NGOs, will implement the evidence-based models to reach entire populations at risk. In the United States, the CDC encourages state health departments and local AIDS service organizations to select specific models that are designated as successful, and an infrastructure for translating the research into practice has developed. Local program implementers are expected either to adopt these models or to provide evaluation evidence that their own activities are effective in preventing HIV transmission (51,52). Both government (93) and private organizations (98) have been careful about the criteria for effectiveness of the models they endorse, and while they may sometimes err on the side of inclusion, their criteria are still reasonable. Although a similar process of dissemination is under way in other areas of prevention and medical care, it is not mandatory for programs in those areas to adopt evidence-based practices (99–101). By serving as gatekeeper, funding organizations in HIV prevention set an important example for other areas of public health. And as we will show, HIV prevention is poised to contribute a key improvement in evaluating the translation process.

The Myth of Exact Replication and the Search for Valid Variation

Evaluation research on the translation of models to practice takes increased prominence in HIV prevention concurrently with other areas of health promotion (99),
behavioral medicine (100), and medical care (101). However, the urgency and
scope of dissemination in HIV prevention are forcing a major improvement in
evaluation of this area: ways to evaluate "valid variation" in the evidence-based
models.

Public health and behavioral health researchers make a mistake when they
equate translation of evidence-based models with the ideal of exact replication.
As noted by the *Harvard Business Review*, "There's no such thing as an exact
copy of a complex organizational activity" (102: 68). The literature on management (102), diffusion of innovations (103), medical care quality improvement
(101), and evaluation in other policy sectors (28) all indicate that practitioners
"reinvent" the models at their own locations (70). In HIV prevention efforts they
are often compelled to do so, because their resources, staffing, settings, and populations are so different from the originals. If nothing else, variations in cultural
dynamics force the adaptation of HIV prevention models to meet unique local
circumstances (104).

The myth of exact replication creates substantial mischief for health promotion programs and their evaluation in general. Behavioral researchers adhere to
the ideal of "treatment with fidelity" and strive to eliminate variation through a
uniform protocol. They tend to view any site-level variations as nuisance variables to be controlled or ignored (105). However, behavioral scientists are working with open systems, not petri dishes. At the point of model transfer, they are
no longer dealing with evaluation of efficacy (controlled conditions) but effectiveness, which addresses real-world conditions. While "treatment with fidelity"
is important for efficacy trials, it requires some basic reassessment when evidence-based models are adopted by HIV prevention practitioners.

Health departments, NGOs, and CBOs often tell the behavioral scientists that
they simply cannot do interventions precisely "by the book" (106,107). Often
their adaptation of prevention interventions is treated as an unacceptable departure from "fidelity" (108), and the researchers frame the problem as a lack of capacity to conduct evidence-based prevention (109,110). There is no question that
many CBOs, NGOs, and health departments do, indeed, need increased capacity to implement proven HIV prevention interventions (111), and this is the case
for other public health programs as well (99,100). However, lack of capacity is
not the entire answer to the problem of variation. Because the models must be
reinvented to meet local needs and circumstances, it would be better to carefully
monitor the ways in which essential components of intervention are modified and
to assess the result. "Valid variation" is an urgent matter for empirical test, not
simply the judgment of the original model developer.

HIV's Contributions to Understanding Valid Variation: New Methods for External Validity

The problem of valid variation is one of external validity—our ability to generalize about the evidence base (28,82). External validity involves replication, preferably with deliberate variation along four dimensions: the population under study; the intervention; the study methods; and the setting, culture, context, and era in which the study takes place (28,82,112). Evaluation in HIV prevention provides some excellent models to increase external validity. For example, in the AIDS Community Demonstration Projects, a core of behavioral and social marketing principles was systematically adapted to the needs of five very different kinds of people at risk (19). More recently, valid variation has been guided by behavioral and program theory and by the use of templates for implementation (102). In an award-winning evaluation, Miller and her colleagues at the Gay Men's Health Crisis of New York City extended the evidence base for a model employing natural opinion leaders within the gay bar scene (60,113). The systematic variation concerned populations (gay prostitutes and their clients in "hustler" bars of New York City, rather than gay men in small cities). In addition, the intervention differed from the original according to a careful template: training scripts and session sequencing were adapted to the lifestyle of gay prostitutes. Most significant for evaluation methods, these differences were monitored closely through process evaluation, both for quality control and to validate the variation by replicating the outcomes.

HIV evaluation is in an excellent position to do more in this area, with beneficial effects on health promotion generally. Evaluation can capitalize on the widespread adoption of evidence-based models to enrich our understanding of how models are modified. If acceptable, these modifications should be rigorously tested, retained as part of craft knowledge, and widely shared with the many organizations coping with similar problems. If the modifications are unacceptable, these conclusions should also be shared widely, as a quality control mechanism. Evaluators of HIV prevention efforts are in an excellent position to develop the knowledge base on valid variation, because of the recent growth in local evaluation capacity.

Creation of Evaluation Capacity

The Centers for Disease Control and Prevention is the U.S. government's lead agency in HIV prevention. Throughout the epidemic, the CDC has provided state and local health departments and CBOs with technical assistance and with personnel and financial support to evaluate HIV prevention (114,115). The CDC HIV Prevention Strategic Plan through 2005 will accomplish its evaluation objectives through collaborative partnerships with other federal agencies and with state and local organizations (116). In its guidance to state and local health departments for HIV prevention activities, the CDC has recently implemented an extensively revised system of evaluation schema (52).

This creation of state and local capacity for evaluation in HIV prevention is probably the largest such effort in U.S. public health history. The evaluation guidelines aim primarily for accountability, but also for program improvement (52). As the nation's prevention agency, the CDC acknowledges that evaluation capacity is being expanded in the face of relatively limited resources, competing demands upon those resources, and a relative scarcity of qualified evaluators in many localities. Quite correctly, the CDC is relying on moral suasion and self-interest to convince funded organizations that evaluation will help meet the common goal of HIV prevention (117). Although street-level HIV prevention workers express considerable cynicism about evaluation, there is also evidence that some organizations are using these systems for their intended purposes (117). In these respects, the national HIV prevention evaluation system is similar to those seen in education and community mental health programs (118,119). Because these systems cannot be audited adequately, the validity of the information must be maintained in other ways. It is very clear that high-quality, decentralized evaluation systems require the buy-in and utilization of data by the local programs (120).

These new developments in HIV prevention evaluation have crystallized the idea of capacity-building for local evaluation, a concept rarely addressed directly in the past (121). This occurs at a time when professional evaluation societies are proliferating internationally. The American Evaluation Association (URL: www.eval.org) lists sixteen links to societies as diverse as the African Evaluation Association and the Walloon Evaluation Society, but not others, such as the Indonesian or Japanese associations.

Key to the idea of evaluation capacity is the search for information that is useful and relevant to the sponsoring organizations. This poses a challenge, since the information that is viewed as valid and pertinent at the community level and across cultures is not necessarily the same as the information viewed as valid by social scientists and funding agencies (12,122,123). The idea of different "ways of knowing" is relatively new for public health, although some community-based health promotion researchers have addressed it in as yet a fairly confined sphere of influence (44,47). A mix of evaluation information is probably needed, some of which will be valid for local stakeholders, and some valid for federal decision makers. Also, local evaluation capacity has to rely on the development of measures that are reasonably inexpensive, are optimally useful for program improvement, and do not impose major response burden on the organizations (67,68). To that end, HIV evaluators at the national and international levels are striving to create indicator systems that could be cheaply employed at the local level (124,125). Performance measurement is currently being extended to HIV prevention as well (126). New developments in HIV prevention, such as the ability to detect new infections, are likely to improve the relevance and specificity of such indicators over time (127).

Evaluation of Established HIV Prevention Programs: Summary of Contributions

The special pressures of HIV prevention produced advances in cost-utility analyses and stimulated more public health professionals outside of HIV, to use cost-utility analysis. Public health could benefit by emulating other examples set by HIV prevention, such as the unique quality control safeguards, based on evaluation evidence, that facilitate use of effective HIV prevention models. Also, opportunities are abundant to improve the external validity (generalization) of the evidence based models. Yet the most important contribution of widespread HIV prevention programs is undoubtedly the increase in evaluation capacity, at all levels of government, and within CBOs and NGOs.

Acknowledgments

We thank Charles Collins, David Cotton, Michael Dennis, Donna Higgins, Steven Isaacs, and Harvey Siegal for their suggestions and guidance.

References

Authors' note: several references were originally published long before HIV. In these cases, original publication dates are noted in brackets.

1. Shadish WR, Cook TD, and Leviton LC: *Foundations of Program Evaluation: Theorists and Their Theories.* Sage, Newbury Park, Ca., 1991.
2. Leviton LC and Hughes EFX: Research on the utilization of evaluations: a review and synthesis. *Eval Rev* 5: 525–547, 1981.
3. Leviton LC and Boruch RF: Contributions of evaluation to education programs and policy. *Eval Rev* 7: 563–598, 1983.
4. Coyle SL, Boruch RF, and Turner CF (eds.): *Evaluating AIDS Prevention Programs.* National Academy Press, Washington, DC, 1989.
5. Sechrest L (ed.): *Health Services Research Methodology: A Focus on AIDS.* (PHS) 89–3439. National Center for Health Services Research, Rockville, MD, 1989.
6. Azjen I and Fishbein M: *Understanding Attitudes and Predicting Social Behavior.* Prentice Hall, Englewood Cliffs, NJ, 1997 [first published 1980].
7. Prochaska JO, Redding CA, Harlow LL, Rossi JS, and Velicer WF: The transtheoretical model of change and HIV prevention: a review. *Health Educ Q* 21: 471–486, 1994.
8. Terry DJ, Gallois C, and McCamish M: *The Theory of Reasoned Action: Its Application to AIDS-Preventive Behavior* (International Series in Experimental Social Psychology, Vol 28). Routledge, New York, 1994.
9. Centers for Disease Control and Prevention: Framework for program evaluation in public health. *Morb Mortal Wkly Rep* 48 (RR-11): 1–40, 1999.

10. Cronbach LJ, Ambron SR, Dornbusch SM, Hess RD, Hornik RC, Phillips DC, Walker DF, and Weiner SS: *Toward Reform of Program Evaluation.* Jossey-Bass, San Francisco, 1980.

11. Gibney L: HIV prevention in developing countries: Tenets of behavioral and biomedical approaches. In Gibney L, DiClemente RJ, and Vermund SH (eds.): *Preventing HIV in Developing Countries: Biomedical and Behavioral Approaches.* Kluwer, New York, 1999, pp. 1–7.

12. Van der Meer FB: Evaluation and the social construction of impacts. *Evaluation* 5: 387–406, 1999.

13. Allen SA, Karita E, N'Gandu N, and Tichacek A: The evolution of voluntary testing and counseling as an HIV prevention strategy. In Gibney L, DiClemente RJ, and Vermund SH (eds.): *Preventing HIV in Developing Countries: Biomedical and Behavioral Approaches.* Kluwer, New York, 1999, pp. 87–108.

14. Dallabetta G, Serwadda D, and Mugrditchian D: Controlling other sexually transmitted diseases. In Gibney L, DiClemente RJ, and Vermund SH (eds.): *Preventing HIV in Developing Countries: Biomedical and Behavioral Approaches.* Kluwer, New York, 1999, pp. 109–136.

15. O'Reilly KR, Msiska R, Mouli VC, and Islam M: Behavioral interventions in developing nations. In Gibney L, DiClemente RJ, and Vermund SH (eds.): *Preventing HIV in Developing Countries: Biomedical and Behavioral Approaches.* Kluwer, New York, 1999, pp. 136–154.

16. Scriven M: *Evaluation Thesaurus*, 4th ed. Sage, Newbury Park, CA, 1991 [first edition 1977].

17. Rossi PH, Freeman HE, and Lipsey MW: *Evaluation: A Systematic Approach*, 6th ed. Sage, Thousand Oaks, CA, 1999 [first edition 1978].

18. Leviton LC and Schuh RG: Evaluation of outreach as a program element. *Eval Rev* 15: 420–440, 1991.

19. Centers for Disease Control and Prevention: Community-level prevention of Human Immunodeficiency Virus Infection among high-risk populations: the AIDS Community Demonstration Projects. *Morb Mortal Wkly Rep* 45 (RR-6): 1–24, 1996.

20. Hein, K: Aligning science with politics and policy in HIV prevention. *Science* 280: 1905–1906, 1998.

21. Kann L, Brener ND, and Allensworth DD: Health education: results from the School Health Policies and Programs Study 2000. *J School Health* 71: 266–278, 2001.

22. Holtgrave DR (ed.): *Handbook of Economic Evaluation of HIV Prevention Programs.* Plenum, New York, 1998.

23. Campbell DT and Stanley JC: *Experimental and Quasi-Experimental Designs for Research.* Houghton-Mifflin, Boston, 1966. [first published 1963].

24. Cook TD and Campbell DT: *Quasi-experimentation.* Rand McNally, Chicago, 1979.

25. Shadish WR, Cook TD, and Campbell DT: *Experimental and Quasi-experimental Designs for Generalized Causal Inference.* Houghton-Mifflin, Boston, 2001.

26. Wholey JS: *Evaluation: Promise and Performance.* Urban Institute, Washington, DC, 1979.

27. Wholey JS, Hatry HP, and Newcomer KE: *Handbook of Practical Program Evaluation.* Jossey-Bass, San Francisco, 1994.

28. Cronbach LJ: *Designing Evaluations of Educational and Social Programs.* Jossey-Bass, San Francisco, 1982.

29. Stake RE: The countenance of educational evaluation. *Teachers College Rec* 68: 523–540, 1967.

30. Patton MQ: *Qualitative Evaluation and Research Methods.* Sage Publications, Thousand Oaks, CA, 1990.

31. Whitmore E: *Understanding and Practicing Participatory Evaluation.* New Directions in Program Evaluation, 80. Jossey-Bass, San Francisco, 1998.

32. Patton MQ: *Utilization-Focused Evaluation.* Sage, Thousand Oaks, CA, 1997 [first edition 1978].

33. Weiss CH: *Evaluation Research: Methods for Assessing Program Effectiveness.* Prentice Hall, Englewood Cliffs, NJ, 1997 [first edition 1972].

34. Suchman EL: *Evaluative Research: Principles and Practice in Public Service and Social Action Programs.* Russell Sage Foundation, New York, 1967.

35. Haddix AC, Teutsch SM, and Shaffer P: *Prevention Effectiveness: A Guide to Decision Analysis and Economic Evaluation.* Oxford University Press, Oxford, 1996.

36. Leviton LC, Collins C, Laird B, and Kratt P: Teaching evaluation using evaluability assessment. *Evaluation* 4: 389–409, 1998.

37. Chen HT and Rossi PH: *Theory-Driven Evaluations.* Sage Publications, Thousand Oaks, CA, 1999.

38. Lipsey MW, Crosse S, Dunkle J, Pollard J, and Stobart G: Evaluation: the state of the art and the sorry state of the science. *New Dir Program Eval* 27: 7–48, 1985.

39. Valdiserri RO (ed.): HIV counseling and testing: its evolving role in HIV prevention. *AIDS Education and Prevention* 9(Suppl. B): 1–118, 1997.

40. Falkson L: An evaluation of policy-related research on citizen participation in municipal health service systems. *Med Care Rev* 33: 156–221, 1976.

41. Systems Research and Development Corporation: *CDC's National Urban Rat Control Program: Background Report and Evaluation of the First Decade.* Author, Washington, D.C., 1980.

42. La Forgia GM: Challenging health service stratification: Social Security–Health Ministry integration in Panama, 1973–1986. Ph.D. diss., University of Pittsburgh, Pittsburgh, Pennsylvania, 1990.

43. Rivkin S: *Community Participation in Maternal and Child Health and Family Planning.* World Health Organization, Geneva, 1990.

44. Parker EA, Eng E, Schulz AJ, and Israel BA: Evaluating community-based health programs that seek to increase community capacity. *New Dir Program Eval* 44: 37–54, 1999.

45. Howell EM, Devaney B, McCormick M, and Raykovich KT: Back to the future: community involvement in the Healthy Start Program. *J Health Politics Policy Law* 23: 291–317, 1998.

46. Turning Point National Program Office: *The Turning Point Initiative: Collaboration for a New Century in Public Health.* Author, Seattle, 2002. URL: www.turning-pointprogram.org.

47. Community Tool Box: *Bringing Solutions to Light.* Author, Lawrence, Kansas, 2002. URL: http://ctb.ukans.edu.

48. National Association of City and County Health Officials: *Mobilizing for Action through Planning and Partnerships (MAPP).* Author, Washington, DC, 2002. URL: www.naccho.org/tools.cfm.

49. National Association of City and County Health Officials: *Assessment Protocol for Excellence in Public Health (APEX-PH).* Author, Washington, DC, 1991. URL: www.naccho.org/tools.cfm.

50. Public Health Practice Office: *The National Public Health Performance Standards*

Program. Centers for Disease Control, Atlanta, 2002. URL: www.phppo.cdc.gov/dphs/nphpsp.

51. Johnson-Masotti AP, Pinkerton SD, Holtgrave DR, Valdiserri RO, and Willingham M: Decision-making in HIV prevention community planning: an integrative review. *J Community Health* 25: 95–112, 2000.

52. National Center for HIV, STD and TB Prevention, Divisions of HIV/AIDS Prevention: *Evaluating CDC-Funded Health Department HIV Prevention Programs,* Vol. 1 and 2. Centers for Disease Control, Atlanta, 2001.

53. Andersen R and Aday LA: Access to medical care in the United States: Realized and potential. *Med Care* 16: 533–546, 1978.

54. Reynolds RA: Improving access to health care among the poor: the neighborhood health center experience. *Milbank Mem Fund Q* 54: 47–82, 1976.

55. Cauffman JG, Wingert WA, Friedman DB, Warburton EA, and Haynes B: Community health aides: How effective are they? *Am J Public Health* 60: 1904–1909, 1970.

56. Moore FI and Stewart JC: Important variables influencing successful use of aides. *Health Serv Rep* 87: 555–561, 1972.

57. Torrey EF, Smith D, and Wise H: The family health worker revisited: a five year follow-up. *Am J Public Health* 63: 71–74, 1973.

58. Packard Foundation: Home visiting: recent program evaluations. *Future Child* 9(1): pp. 1–223, 1999.

59. Groce NE and Reeve ME: Traditional healers and global surveillance strategies for emerging diseases: closing the gap. *Emerging Infect Dis* 2: 351–353, 1996.

60. Kelly JA, Murphy DA, Sikkema KJ, McAuliffe TL, Roffman RA, Solomon LJ, Winett RA, Kalichman SC, and the Community HIV Prevention Research Collaborative: Randomised, controlled, community-level HIV-prevention intervention for sexual-risk behaviour among homosexual men in U.S. cities. *Lancet* 350: 1500–1505, 1997.

61. Brown B, Beschner G, and the National AIDS Consortium: *At Risk for AIDS: Injection Drug Users and Sexual Partners.* Greenwood Press, Westport, CT, 1993.

62. Greenberg JB and Neumann MS: *What We Have Learned from the AIDS Evaluation of Street Outreach Projects: A Summary Document.* Centers for Disease Control and Prevention, Atlanta, 1998.

63. Siegal HA, Carlson RG, Falck RS, and Wang J: Drug abuse treatment experience and HIV risk behaviors among active drug injectors in Ohio. *Am J Public Health* 85: 105–108, 1995.

64. Miller RL and Solomon EE: Assessing the AIDS-related needs of women in a Brooklyn housing development. In Reviere R, Berkowitz S, Carter CC, and Ferguson CG (eds.): *Needs Assessment: A Practical and Creative Guide for Social Scientists.* Taylor and Francis, London, 1996, pp. 93–119.

65. Lauby JL, Smith PJ, Stark M, Person B, and Adams J: A community-level HIV prevention intervention for inner-city women: results of the women and infants demonstration projects. *Am J Public Health* 90: 216–222, 2000.

66. Cabral RJ, Galavotti C, Gargiullo PM, et al.: Paraprofessional delivery of a theory based HIV prevention counseling intervention for women. *Public Health Rep* 111: 75–82, 1996.

67. Mantell JE, DiVittis AT, and Auerbach MI: *Evaluating HIV Prevention Interventions.* Plenum, New York, 1997.

68. Miller RL and Cassel BJ: Ongoing evaluation in AIDS-service organizations: building meaningful evaluation activities. *J Prev Inter Community* 19: 21–39, 1999.

69. Green LW and Kreuter MW: *Health Promotion Planning: An Educational and Eco-logical Approach.* Mayfield, Palo Alto, CA, 1999 [first edition 1980].
70. Leviton LC: Integrating psychology and public health: challenges and opportunities. *Am Psychol* 51: 42–51, 1996.
71. Brandt AM: *No Magic Bullet: A Social History of Venereal Disease in the United States since 1880.* Oxford University Press, Oxford, 1987.
72. Higgins D, Galavotti C, O'Reilly K, and Sheridan J: Evolution and development of the AIDS Community Demonstration projects. In Corby NH and Wolitski RJ (eds.): *Community HIV Prevention: The Long Beach AIDS Community Demonstration Project.* University Press, California State University, Long Beach, 1997, pp. 5–20.
73. Fishbein M, Triandis HC, Kanfer FH, Becker M, Middlestadt S, and Eichler A: Factors influencing behavior and behavior change. In Baum A, Revenson TA, and Singer JE (eds.): *Handbook of Health Psychology.* Lawrence Erlbaum, Englewood Cliffs, NJ, 2001, pp. 3–18.
74. Schneiderman N, Speers MA, Silva JM, Tomes H, and Gentry JH: *Integrating Behavioral and Social Sciences with Public Health.* American Psychological Association, Washington, DC, 2001.
75. Murray DM: *Design and Analysis of Group-Randomized Trials.* Oxford University Press, New York, 1998.
76. Pinkerton SD, Holtgrave DR, Leviton LC, Wagstaff DA, Cecil H, and Abramson PR: Toward a standardized sexual behavior data collection for HIV prevention effectiveness evaluation. *Am J Health Behav* 22: 259–266, 1998.
77. Schensul JJ and Schensul SL: Ethnographic evaluation of AIDS prevention programs: better data for better programs. *New Dir Program Eval* 46: 51–62, 1990.
78. Higgins DL, O'Reilly K, Tashima N, Crain C, Beeker C, Goldbaum G, Elifson CS, Galavotti C, and Guenther-Grey C: Using formative research to lay the foundation for community level HIV prevention efforts: an example from the AIDS Community Demonstration Projects. *Public Health Rep* 111(suppl): 28–35, 1996.
79. Scrimshaw SCM, Carballo M, Ramos L, and Blair BA: The AIDS Rapid Anthropological Assessment Procedures: a tool for health education planning and evaluation. *Health Educ Q* 18: 111–123, 1991.
80. Scrimshaw SCM and Hurtado E: *Rapid Assessment Procedures for Nutrition and Primary Health Care* (Anthropological Approaches to Improving Programme Effectiveness). UCLA Latin American Center, Los Angeles, 1987.
81. Muhib F, Lin L, Steuve A, Miller RL, Ford W, Johnson W, Smith P, and the Community Intervention Trial for Youth (CITY) Study Team: A venue-based method for sampling hard to reach populations. *Public Health Rep* 116(suppl. 2): 216–222, 2001.
82. Leviton LC: External validity. In Smelser NJ and Baltes PB (eds.): *The International Encyclopedia of the Social and Behavioral Sciences.* Cambridge University Press, Cambridge, 8: 5195–5200, 2001.
83. McAlister A, Puska P, Salonen JT, Tuomilehto J, and Koskela K: Theory and action for health promotion: illustrations from the North Karelia Project. *Am J Public Health* 72: 43–50, 1982.
84. Susser M: The tribulations of trials: interventions in communities [editorial]. *Am J Public Health* 85: 156–158, 1995.
85. St. Lawrence JS and McFarlane M: Research methods in the study of sexual behavior. In Kendall PC, Butcher JN, & Holmbeck GN (eds.): *Handbook of Research Methods in Clinical Psychology*, 2nd ed. Wiley, New York, 1999, pp. 584–615.
86. Laumann EO, Gagnon JH, Michael RT, and Michaels S: *The Social Organization*

of Sexuality: Sexual Practices in the United States. University of Chicago Press, Chicago, 1994.

87. Susser I and Stein Z: Culture, sexuality, and women's agency in the prevention of HIV/AIDS in southern Africa. *Am J Public Health* 90: 1042–1048, 2000.

88. Hatfield E, Rapson RL, and Rapson R: *Love and Sex: Cross-Cultural Perspectives.* Allyn and Bacon, Boston, 1995.

89. McLellan AT, Belding M, McKay JR, Zanis D, and Alterman AI: Can the outcomes research literature inform the search for quality indicators in substance abuse treatment? In Edmunds M, Frank R, Hogan M, McCarty D, Robinson-Beale R, and Weisner C (eds.): *Managing Managed Care: Quality Improvement in Behavioral Health.* National Academy Press, Washington DC, 1997, pp. 271–311.

90. Institute of Medicine, Committee on Community-Based Drug Treatment Research: *Bridging the Gap between Practice and Research.* National Academy Press, Washington, DC, 1998.

91. Hubbard RL, Craddock SG, Flynn PM, Anderson J, and Etheridge RM: Overview of 1-Year Follow-Up Outcomes in the Drug Abuse Treatment Outcome Study (DATOS). *Psychol Addict Behav* 11: 261–278, 1997.

92. O'Connor E: Real-world research: the Clinical Trials Network. *Monit Psychol* 32: 28–29, 2001.

93. Centers for Disease Control and Prevention, Prevention Research Synthesis Project: *Compendium of HIV Prevention Interventions with Evidence of Effectiveness.* CDC, Atlanta, 1999. URL: www.cdc.gov/hiv/pubs/hivcompendium/HIVcompendium.pdf.

94. Kaplan EH: An overview of AIDS modeling. *New Dir Program Eval* 46, 1990, pp. 23–36.

95. Pinkerton SD, Holtgrave DR, and Valdiserri RO: Cost-effectiveness of HIV-prevention skills training for men who have sex with men. *AIDS* 11: 347–357, 1997.

96. Russell LS: *Is Prevention Better Than Cure?* Brookings Institution, Washington, DC, 1985.

97. Weinstein MC and Stason WB: *Hypertension Control: A Policy Perspective.* Harvard University Press, Cambridge, MA, 1976.

98. Card JJ, Niego S, Mallari A, and Farrell WS: The program archive on sexuality, health and adolescence: promising "prevention programs in a box." *Fam Plann Perspect* 28: 210–220, 1996.

99. Glasgow RE, Vogt TM, and Boles SM: Evaluating the public health impact of health promotion interventions: the RE-AIM framework. *Am J Public Health* 89: 1322–1327, 1999.

100. Orleans CT: The challenge of translating research to practice: everything I needed to know I learned from tobacco. Presidential address at the Annual Conference of the Society of Behavioral Medicine, Seattle, March 21–24, 2001.

101. Agency for Health Care Policy and Research: *Annotated Bibliography: Information Dissemination to Health Care Practitioners and Policymakers.* Author, Rockville, MD, 1992.

102. Szulanski G and Winter S: Getting it right the second time. *Harv Business Rev* 80: 62–69, 2002.

103. Rogers EM: *Diffusion of Innovations*, 4th ed. Free Press, New York, 1995 [first edition 1962].

104. Raj A, Mukherjee S, and Leviton L: Insights for HIV prevention from industrialized countries' experiences. In Gibney L, DiClemente RJ, and Vermund SH (eds.): *Pre-*

venting HIV in Developing Countries: Biomedical and Behavioral Approaches. Kluwer, New York, 1999.

105. Leviton LC: Symposium: "Integrating Psychology and Public Health: Theories, Models and Practices." Paper presented at "Public Health in the 21st Century," a joint meeting of the American Psychological Association and the Centers for Disease Control and Prevention, Atlanta, May 9, 1998.

106. Miller RL: Innovation in HIV prevention: organizational and intervention characteristics affecting program adoption. *Am J Community Psychol* 29: 621–642, 2001.

107. DeFranceisco W, Kelly JA, Otto-Salaj L, McAuliffe TL, Somlai AM, Hackl K, Heckman TG, Holtgrave DR, and Rompa DJ: Factors influencing attitudes within AIDS service organizations toward the use of research-based HIV prevention interventions. *AIDS Educ Prev* 11: 72–86, 1999.

108. Kalichman SC, Belcher L, Cherry C, and Williams E: Primary prevention of sexually transmitted HIV infections: transferring behavioral research to community programs. *J Prim Prev* 18: 149–172, 1997.

109. Somlai AM, Kelly JA, Otto-Salaj L, McAuliffe TL, Hackl K, DiFranceisco W, Amick B, Heckman TG, Holtgrave DR, and Rompa DJ: Current HIV prevention activities for women and gay men among 77 ASOs. *J Public Health Manag Pract* 5: 23–33, 1999.

110. Kelly JA, Somlai AM, Otto-Salaj LL, McAuliffe TL, DiFranceisco W, Hackl KL, and Rompa DR: Bridging the gap between science and service: a randomized trial of technical assistance methods to transfer research-based HIV prevention approaches to CBOs. Paper presented at the Global Conference on AIDS, Geneva, Switzerland, July 1998.

111. Miller RL, Bedney BJ, and Guenther-Grey C: Assessing community capacity to provide HIV prevention services: the feasibility, evaluability, sustainability assessment protocol. *Health Promot Pract*, in press.

112. Cook TD: A quasi-sampling theory of the generalization of causal relationships. In Sechrest LB and Scott AG (eds.): Understanding causes and generalizing about them. *New Directions for Program Evaluation* 57: 39–82, 1993.

113. Miller RL, Klotz D, and Eckholdt HM: HIV prevention with male prostitutes and patrons of hustler bars: replication of an HIV preventive intervention. *Am J Community Psychol* 26: 97–131, 1998.

114. Bailey ME: Developing a national HIV/AIDS prevention program through state health departments. *Public Health Rep* 106: 695–701, 1991.

115. Centers for Disease Control and Prevention: *Cooperative Agreements for Human Immunodeficiency Virus (HIV): Prevention Projects Program Announcement and Availability of Funds for Fiscal Year 1993.* Author, Atlanta, 1992.

116. Centers for Disease Control and Prevention: *HIV Prevention Strategic Plan through 2005.* Author, Atlanta, 2001.

117. Collins CB, Lacson R, and Cotton D: building evaluation capacity for health departments. Paper presented at the National HIV Prevention Conference, Atlanta, August 12–15, 2001 (abstract #358, p. 189).

118. Boruch RF, Cordray DS, Pion GM, and Leviton LC: A mandated appraisal of evaluation practices: digest of recommendations to the Congress and the Department of Education. *Educ Res* 10: 10–13, 31, 1981.

119. Landsberg G, Neigher WD, Hammer RJ, Windle C, and Woy JR (eds.): *Evaluation in Practice: A Sourcebook of Program Evaluation Studies from Mental Health Care*

Systems in the United States. (DHEW Publication No. ADM 78–763). U. S. Government Printing Office, Washington, DC, 1979.

120. Leviton LC: Capacity-building for evaluation of HIV prevention. Paper presented at the first Centers for Disease Control and Prevention HIV Prevention Evaluation meeting, Atlanta, June 19, 2001.

121. Cotton D and Milstein B: *Working Draft: Defining Concepts for the Presidential Stand on Building Evaluation Capacity.* American Evaluation Association. 2000. URL: www.eval.org/eval2000/presstrand.htm.

122. Solomon EE and Miller RL: Developing collaborative relationships: the Brooklyn Women's Project. In Sayad J (ed.): *Models of Collaborative Research.* American Public Health Association, Washington, DC, 2001.

123. Feurstein MT: *Partners in Evaluation: Evaluating Development and Community Programmes with Participants.* MacMillian, London, 1986.

124. Mertens T, Carael M, Sato P, Cleland J, Ward H, and Smith GD: Prevention indicators for evaluating the progress of national AIDS programmes. *AIDS* 8: 1359–1369, 1994.

125. Page-Shafer K, Kim A, Norton P, Rugg D, Heitgerd J, Katz MH, McFarland W, and the HIV Prevention Indicators Field Collaborative: Evaluating national HIV prevention indicators: a case study in San Francisco. *AIDS* 14: 2015–2026, 2000.

126. Hatry H: *Performance Measurement: Getting Results.* Urban Institute, Washington, DC, 1999.

127. Janssen RS, Satten GA, Stramer SL, Bhupat DR, O'Brien TR, Weiblen BJ, Hecht FM, Jack N, Cleghorn FR, Kahn JO, Chesney MA, and Busch MP: New testing strategy to detect early HIV-1 infection for use in incidence estimates and for clinical and prevention purposes. *JAMA* 280: 42–48, 1998.

9

The Evolving Impact of HIV/AIDS on Global Health

PETER LAMPTEY, KRISTEN RUCKSTUHL,
AND WILLARD CATES, JR.

For much of its history to date, HIV/AIDS has been viewed primarily as a public health issue. With the increasing realization of its vast impact on social, economic, and political systems, however, the disease is emerging as a major factor in global development strategies. As a result, HIV/AIDS is commanding much more attention from world leaders. In 2001, the U.N. Secretary-General Kofi Annan made HIV/AIDS his personal priority and challenged his peers to "define AIDS . . . as a threat to our common future and as a test of our common humanity" (1). And on June 25–27, 2001, the United Nations General Assembly held a Special Session (UNGASS) that brought together key heads and representatives of states and governments and representatives from non-governmental organizations (NGOs), the private sector, activists, and foundations to address the global HIV/AIDS epidemic.

The UNGASS meeting helped demonstrate that HIV/AIDS is a global crisis and that urgent and unprecedented action involving unique partnerships is needed to stop it (2). This meeting addressed the many facets of the HIV/AIDS epidemic, including human rights issues and the public health, social, and economic effects, as well as the developmental impact of the epidemic. A global HIV/AIDS and health fund with a target of $9 billion was created to support integrated approaches to prevention, care, support, and treatment. The establishment of this fund helped refocus attention not only on HIV/AIDS, but also on two other important threats to international health, tuberculosis (TB) and malaria.

The participants produced a 103 point Declaration of Commitment to prevent HIV spread by enhancing political will and intensifying national, regional, and international attention. The world leaders at UNGASS expressed a deep concern that the global HIV/AIDS epidemic, through its devastating effects, constitutes a true global emergency. Their statement highlighted several key themes:

• Strong leadership is needed at all societal levels.
• Prevention must be the main global response.
• Care, support, and treatment are fundamental elements of an effective response.
• Human rights, especially empowerment of women, are essential to reducing vulnerability to HIV/AIDS.
• Respect for the rights of people living with HIV/AIDS is crucial.

These declarations and actions of UNGASS are not only critical for the successful prevention, care, and treatment of HIV/AIDS, but they will also have a profound effect on other dimensions of global health, including public health practice, the social and economic environment, human rights, and reducing the vulnerability of women to health and other societal threats.

Our chapter will address the evolving impact of HIV/AIDS on the broader global health agenda.

Global Burden of Disease

According to the most recent UNAIDS statistics, by the end of the year 2001, an estimated 40 million people worldwide were living with HIV or AIDS. Of this number, the vast majority were living in resource-poor settings; more than 28.1 million, or seven out of ten, were living in sub-Saharan Africa (Figure 9–1) (3).

Globally, by the end of 2001, HIV/AIDS had caused an estimated 25 million adult and child deaths. Of this number, 19.3 million deaths (almost 80 percent) were in Africa, 3.4 million in South and Southeast Asia, 590,000 in Latin America, 448,000 in North America, 272,000 in the Caribbean, and 58,000 in Eastern Europe and Central Asia. And, the number of new HIV/AIDS infections in developing countries continues to increase. In 2001, an estimated 5 million (3.4 million of those in Africa) adults and children were newly infected with HIV (Figure 9–2) (3).

Globally, it is estimated that there are some 14,000 new HIV infections a day, over 95 percent of them occurring in developing countries. Of the new infections, about 2,000 are in children under 15 years, and 12,000 of them are in adults aged 15 to 49 years. Almost half of all new infections are among women, and about 50 percent are in young adults aged 15 to 24 years (3).

Worldwide, the route of HIV transmission varies by region (4). In Africa, het-

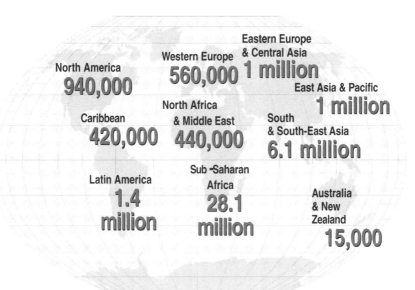

Total: 40 million

FIGURE 9–1. Adults and children estimated to be living with HIV/AIDS as of end of 2001. *Source*: UNAIDS/WHO 2001.

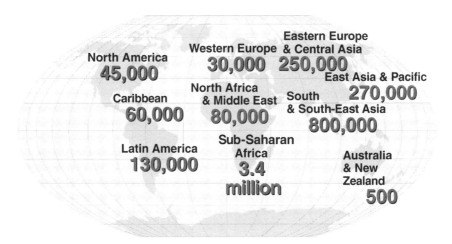

Total: 5 million

FIGURE 9–2. Estimated number of adults and children newly infected with HIV during 2001. *Source*: UNAIDS/WHO 2001.

erosexual contact accounts for most of the spread. Using HIV serosurveys of women attending prenatal clinics as a proxy for sexual transmission (Figure 9–3), countries in sub-Saharan Africa have suffered rapidly rising HIV prevalence rates. In addition, in Africa, transfusion of contaminated blood and mother-to-child transmission contribute a sizeable proportion of infections.

In Latin America, most infections are transmitted through men having sex with men (MSM) and injection drug use (IDU), but heterosexual transmission is rising. In the Caribbean, heterosexual spread is the dominant mode, but MSM transmission continues to play an important role. Heterosexual contact and IDU are the two main modes of HIV transmission in South and Southeast Asia. In Eastern Europe and Central Asia, IDUs are the group with the fastest rising HIV incidence.

Demographic and Social Impact of HIV/AIDS

The worldwide demographic and social impact of the HIV/AIDS pandemic is devastating. In many African countries, population growth rates have plummeted, and the age composition is changing. Figure 9–4 illustrates the dramatic changes in the population of Botswana as a result of HIV/AIDS.

In countries with high HIV prevalence and relatively low fertility rates (i.e., number of live births per 1,000 women of child bearing ages), population levels have stabilized. In Zimbabwe, for example, a country with a fertility rate of 4, the population growth rate is now below 1 percent (5). According to recent national census estimates, some of the countries with the highest HIV prevalence

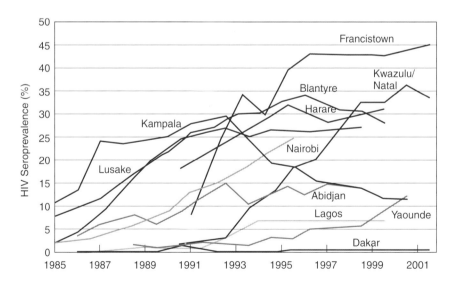

FIGURE 9–3. HIV seroprevalence for pregnant women in selected urban areas in Africa, 1985–2001. *Note*: Includes infection from HIV-1 and/or HIV-2. *Source*: US Census Bureau, HIV/AIDS Surveillance Data Base, 2002.

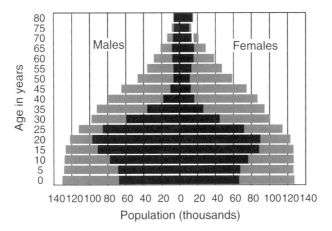

FIGURE 9–4. Projected population structure with and without the AIDS epidemic, Botswana, 2020. Black indicates projected population structure in 2020; light gray indicates deficits due to AIDS. *Source*: US Census Bureau, World Population Profile 2000.

will experience a negative population growth within the next three to four years (6).

In many parts of the developing world, gains in life expectancy achieved over the past half-century have been reversed by the HIV/AIDS pandemic. A Zimbabwean in the year 2001 can expect to live to age 39, down from 71 years a decade ago (6). In Zimbabwe, infant mortality without AIDS is estimated at 30 infant deaths per 1,000 live births. Instead, with HIV/AIDS, infant mortality is more than twice that level (7). Unfortunately, this pattern of rapidly decreasing life expectancies as a result of increasing infant and child mortality is the norm in most sub-Saharan African countries with high HIV prevalence rates (Figure 9–5). The deterioration of life expectancy rates brought about by HIV/AIDS is expected to continue throughout the developing world for at least the next decade.

The social impact of the HIV/AIDS epidemic in the developing world is equally grim. HIV/AIDS has been responsible for a profound weakening, and in some cases, a breakdown of a variety of societal institutions, including educational, civil service, armed forces, and health services (8). Countries hard hit by the epidemic are facing limitations of private-sector growth, as well as an overall destruction of social capital, including the production and knowledge bases of societies. In particular, the most productive human resources are directly affected by HIV/AIDS. The human development index (HDI) measures a combination of countries' gross domestic product, adult literacy, and life expectancy. The United Nations Development Programme has estimated that in South Africa, by 2010, their national HDI would be 15 percent lower due to HIV/AIDS (8).

HIV/AIDS has also had devastating effects at the individual household level. For example, the number of AIDS orphans estimated by UNAIDS at the end of

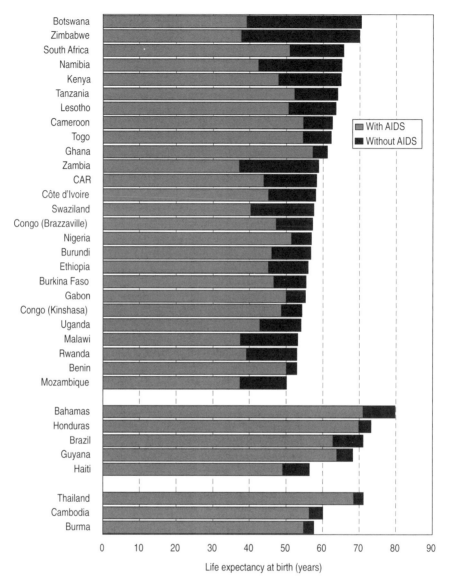

FIGURE 9–5. Life expectancy with and without the AIDS epidemic in 2000. *Source*: U.S. Census Bureau, International Data Base and unpublished tables.

1999 was 13 million (3). By 2010, this number is expected to triple. Children orphaned by HIV/AIDS who live without parental support and protection, lose opportunities for nutrition, health care, and shelter. School attendance among orphans is lower than those with living parents. In the Central African Republic, as of 2001, the national school attendance average was 60 percent, but only 39 percent among orphans (9). The HIV/AIDS challenges faced by children, families, and their communities are interrelated to all sectors of development.

Health-care facilities in some parts of the world have been overrun with HIV/AIDS patients (10). In South Africa, some hospitals devote 80 percent of their beds to caring for HIV-infected persons, and in some rural areas hospitals are 25 percent over capacity. Moreover, this health-care situation will only continue to worsen, given the estimated five- to six-year incubation period of HIV in Africa (11). The flood of HIV patients seen in 2001 represents those infected in the mid-1990s; HIV prevalence rates of 2001 are more than three times as high as those of the 1990s in South Africa. In addition, patients with conditions other than HIV are suffering; elective surgeries have been cancelled, and patients receive inadequate medical and nursing care because the demands posed by HIV/AIDS are so great. Triage responsibilities have sapped existing staff resources, and the need to ration scarce health care resources has created "ethical nightmares" (12). The HIV situation has cast a long shadow on the already constrained health systems of resource-poor countries.

Impact of HIV/AIDS on Economic Development

HIV/AIDS affects economic development at multiple levels. At the household level, HIV/AIDS has changed family composition, its earning potential, its consumption capabilities, and its overall psychosocial well-being. Financial constraints are exacerbated as extended family members, neighbors, and friends take AIDS orphans and other vulnerable children into their households. Families must pay not only for symptomatic treatment of opportunistic infections associated with HIV disease but also for funeral expenses when their loved ones die (6). In Rwanda in 2000, annual per capita health expenditure from households with a person living with AIDS was $63 compared to the average of $3; fewer than 30 percent of households were able to cover the costs of health care with their own resources (13). Household production is greatly decreased and household savings are used up as a result of HIV/AIDS. In Zimbabwe, in households with an AIDS death, household production was reduced by 60 percent (14).

At the private-sector level, the effects of HIV/AIDS are also acutely felt. Additional business costs associated with the disease are the result of increases in absenteeism, labor turnover, recruitment and training investments, insurance and health-care costs, and family pensions (15). Because of increasing AIDS mortality among the segment of adults most active in the labor force, HIV/AIDS has had a profound negative effect on business output in many nations of the developing world. According to Harare-based SafAIDS, in Zimbabwe, by the year 2015, the labor force will be one-sixth smaller (16). Anglo-American, a South African mining company, reported that in 2001 40 percent of lost work time in Zimbabwe was a direct result of HIV/AIDS (16). Additionally, in Zimbabwe, communal farming output has dropped by 50 percent between 1995 and 2000 due in large part to HIV/AIDS (16). Production losses due to HIV/AIDS at a tea estate in Malawi were said to be more than 3 percent of the gross product in 1995–1996 (17).

In summary, the global burden of HIV/AIDS has already transformed many societies. Even worse, the HIV epidemic appears to be gaining demographic and economic momentum.

Successful Strategies to Prevent HIV/AIDS in the Developing World

Despite the devastating impact of HIV/AIDS and its continued spread in most of the developing world, several countries, including Thailand, Senegal, Uganda, Cambodia, and Zambia, have reported meaningful declines in the prevalence of HIV among various population groups. We describe here some of the key approaches that have been successfully used to prevent HIV in developing countries.

100 Percent Condom Promotion Program in Thailand

In Thailand, the first program for "100 percent condom use" was initiated in 1989 in Ratchaburi Province (18). The program promoted condom use during commercial sexual encounters in brothels and other settings. Local statutes were developed, which required the owners of entertainment establishments to enforce condom use in any sexual encounter taking place in their facilities. Further, sex workers were instructed to refuse sex to any customer who would not use a condom. In Ratchaburi, reported condom use increased, leading to decreases in the incidence of sexually transmitted infections (STIs) and the prevalence of HIV (18).

Starting in 1991, the 100 percent condom approach became a nationwide program in Thailand. By the end of the second year of the national program, condom-use rates in commercial sex facilities had increased to as high as 95 percent of all sexual encounters, and the incidence of STIs had decreased from 6.5 infections per 1,000 population to 2.01 per 1,000, over a three-year period (18).

UNAIDS supported an external evaluation of the national 100 percent condom use program and concluded that the program likely prevented over 200,000 cases of STIs annually and more than 2 million HIV infections in Thailand between 1989 and 1995. The reduction in high-risk sexual behavior and the corresponding declines in HIV and other STIs in young adults in Thailand has been impressive (18). The 100 percent condom use program has been successfully replicated in other countries as well, most notably in Cambodia (16).

STI Management in HIV Prevention

An "epidemiological synergy" exists between HIV infection and other STIs (19). Each may enhance the transmission or alter the manifestations of the other, re-

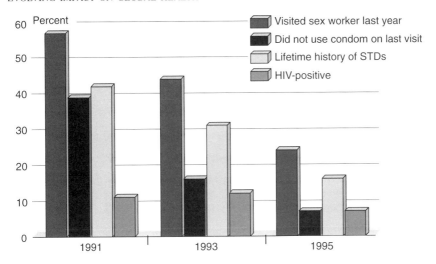

FIGURE 9–6. Sexual behavior, STDs and HIV in 21-year-old men, Northern Thailand, 1991–1995. *Source*: Nelson et al., *New England Journal of Medicine*, 1996; 335:297–303.

sulting in an explosive, mutually reinforcing spiral of infection. Clinical and laboratory evidence shows that STIs facilitate sexual HIV transmission; likewise, HIV-induced immunodeficiency alters the natural history and therapeutic response of other STIs and thus creates bi-directional interactions between these effects. In sum, other STIs are biologically, behaviorally, and epidemiologically inextricably linked to HIV (20).

To assess the population-level impact of STI treatment on HIV transmission, several major community-level evaluations have been conducted. One trial, in the Mwanza District of Tanzania, documented that continuous provision of improved STI services reduced the acquisition of HIV infection (21). A second trial in the Rakai District of Uganda, using intermittent mass STI treatment of the general population, however, found no difference in the incidence of HIV infection between the intervention and the comparison communities (22,23). A third investigation in Lesedi, South Africa, was comprised of presumptive treatment of sex workers with azithromycin, regardless of their symptoms. After nearly a year, rates of gonorrhea and chlamydia had fallen more than 50 percent among the sex workers, and genital ulcer disease decreased by 75 percent. Among clients, symptomatic STDs declined as well, disproportionately so in those served by sex workers participating in the study (24). While the effects of STI treatment on HIV transmission were not measured directly in the Lesedi study, given the epidemiological synergy mentioned, the treatment of STIs may slow down the reinforcing spiral of co-infection between HIV and STIs.

Important lessons were learned from the studies (25–27). First, provision of continuous STI treatment appeared more successful than intermittent or episodic

STI service delivery in terms of HIV prevention. Second, the stage of an HIV epidemic may be crucial in terms of mediating the impact of STI treatment on HIV transmission. At the time of the first trial, Mwanza was experiencing a relatively early HIV epidemic, with community HIV prevalence of 4 percent, whereas the Rakai study took place in one of the world's most mature epidemics, with a community HIV prevalence of approximately 16 percent (21,23). Third, HIV incidence may be disproportionately affected by levels of symptomatic STIs in which shedding is increased, while STI incidence may be more closely related to the prevalence of asymptomatic STIs among the population. Fourth, targeting the highest frequency transmitters for STI treatment may magnify the effect on HIV spread. Fifth and finally, the effect of treating STIs on HIV viral load and viral shedding must be better defined through additional clinical studies (28,29).

Voluntary HIV Counseling and Testing

Fewer than 10 percent of the people living with HIV and AIDS in developing countries are aware of their HIV status. Poor access and availability of voluntary counseling and testing (VCT) services, lack of treatment services, widespread stigma and discrimination against those infected, and the cost of the services have contributed to the low levels of testing. Advocacy for HIV testing as a prevention strategy has also been hampered by the lack of efficacy data (30).

From April 1995 to April 1997, a randomized controlled trial of VCT was conducted by Family Health International, UNAIDS, and the World Health Organization in collaboration with researchers from the United States, Kenya, Tanzania, and Trinidad. In this study, individual and couple participants were randomly assigned to receive either VCT or basic health information (HI). Individual men assigned to VCT reported reduced unprotected intercourse with non-primary partners by 35 percent, compared to a 13 percent decrease by the men assigned to HI. Women in the VCT group reported a 38 percent reduction in unprotected intercourse versus a 17 percent reduction by women assigned to HI. Within the VCT group, individuals diagnosed with HIV were more likely than uninfected individuals to reduce unprotected intercourse with primary partners. Couples in which one or both members were diagnosed with HIV were more likely to reduce unprotected intercourse with each other than couples in which both members were uninfected. At follow-up, when the control group receiving HI was offered VCT, 90 percent wanted to be tested. Finally, the study demonstrated that VCT is a cost-effective intervention for behavior change (30).

Simplified Antiretroviral Prophylaxis for the Prevention of
Mother-to-Child Transmission

In the more developed countries, substantial reductions in mother-to-child transmission (MTCT) of HIV have occurred during the 1990s (31,32). This has been primarily due to the widespread application of a three-part zidovudine regimen to interrupt both prenatal and intrapartum HIV transmission. However, in re-source-poor settings, this approach is both too expensive and too complex to use. A 1999 international clinical trial demonstrated that transmission of HIV from mother to infant could be reduced by up to 50 percent by administration of a short-course antiretroviral treatment during labor and delivery (33). An in-expensive regimen of nevirapine, a potent non-nucleoside reverse transcriptase inhibitor, has shown particular promise. Difficulties in administering the drug are minimized with this regimen, since it consists of a single dose to the mother, intrapartum, and a single dose to the infant, twenty-four to seventy-two hours after birth. Evidence to date shows long-term resistance to nevirapine does not occur with this single dose. Thus, the risk of sexual transmission of nevirapine-resistant virus is likely low, and prophylaxis with this drug would likely remain effective for interruption of intrapartum transmission in future pregnancies.

While this two-dose intrapartum/neonatal nevirapine regimen offers hope, the global challenge is to translate the regimen into effective community-based pub-lic health programs. The absence of widespread antenatal programs, as well as the limitations of VCT access, has shifted attention to the best way of adminis-tering this drug at the population level. In some settings where HIV prevalence is high, it appears more cost effective to routinely administer nevirapine to all women in labor rather than to test and treat only those who are found to be HIV positive (34).

Moreover, with the effectiveness of intrapartum antiretrovirals demonstrated, the focus of preventing mother to child transmission has now broadened to in-clude the breastfeeding interval (31). Data have shown that approximately 10 per-cent of infants who do not become infected by their mothers at the time of de-livery acquire HIV through breastfeeding (35). Infants who receive formula feeding are not exposed to further infection. In a clinical trial in Kenya, formula feeding by cup reduced postnatal transmission by 44 percent; moreover, 75 per-cent of breastfeeding transmission occurred during the first six months of life. Because of this, early weaning alone would not eliminate most HIV transmis-sion during this interval (36).

HIV/AIDS' Influence on Global Public Health

Spurred by reports from the International AIDS Conference in Durban, South Africa, in July 2000, world leaders have increasingly recognized the predom-inance of HIV/AIDS as a macro determinant of global progress. The remain-der of the chapter will address how HIV/AIDS has acted as a catalyst to the overall field of global health and has brought about improvements in broader global arenas.

Impact of HIV on Other Emerging Infectious Diseases

As a result of improved communication and transportation, the world has become a "global village." Furthermore, increased migration, including rapid growth of urban populations and cross-border travel, environmental degradation, and the deterioration of public health infrastructures—all facilitate the spread of infectious diseases (37). The immune dysfunction caused by HIV has led to increased susceptibility of HIV-infected persons worldwide to infectious diseases such as TB. Some 40 percent of HIV-infected individuals have tuberculosis (TB), and it is the leading cause of death in AIDS patients worldwide. TB is on the rise around the globe, due in part to its close association with HIV infection. In addition, there is an increasing spread of TB from individuals with TB/HIV co-infection to non-HIV-infected individuals. The incidence of other opportunistic infections, such as oral candidiasis and cryptococcal meningitis, has also increased as a result of AIDS.

One of the lasting global consequences of the HIV experience is an increased awareness of emerging infectious diseases. Emerging diseases of global concern include drug-resistant TB, drug-resistant malaria, Ebola hemorrhagic fever, a new form of cholera, hemolytic uraemic syndrome, hepatitis C and hepatitis E, Legionnaires' disease, and Lyme disease (38). Lessons learned from HIV are being applied at the national and international levels to improve policies, capacity for research, training, surveillance, response, and prevention of these emerging and reemerging infectious diseases (39).

These lessons include an awareness of the need for increased global cooperation to stem the spread of infectious diseases so as to mitigate the impact on social, economic, military, and political structures. Also critical is the mobilization and involvement of affected communities and multiple sectors in governmental and civil society.

Impact of HIV/AIDS on National and International Security

The HIV/AIDS pandemic has come to be seen as a potential threat to both national and international security. The demographic/political effects of the virus create a danger to the world's stability (37). As HIV/AIDS ravages developing countries, the opportunity for "political polarization" between rich and poor nations is heightened, thus threatening a disruption of global political dynamics. Dwindling resources can fuel further instability within already immature political systems and potentially diminish the capacity of democratization efforts in these countries.

HIV/AIDS affects at least five levels of security: personal, economic, communal, national, and international (40). At the personal level, as more adults become fatally ill, families and communities break apart. In the economic realm, experts predict that an adult HIV prevalence rate of 10 percent can reduce national income by as much as one-third (3). Communally, AIDS depletes the human resources necessary to lead societies—civil servants, teachers, health-care professionals, and police. Rates of infection can be high in military forces, creating a loss of healthy soldiers. A year 2000 study by the U.S. Pentagon revealed that HIV prevalence among African militaries ranges from 10 to 60 percent. These high statistics—together with anecdotal reports stating that infected officers and soldiers are more likely to engage in high-risk behavior and criminal behavior on the battlefield and are less interested in peace negotiations–have serious ramifications on a nation's ability to both defend itself and act as an effective partner in global security (41).

Nationally, civil disruptions of productivity could lead to internal conflict, which might weaken police and military systems, conceivably leading to civil war. In a January 2000 report, the U.S. government and the National Intelligence Council announced that they considered HIV/AIDS and other infectious diseases as threats to national security and that protecting the health and safety of U.S. citizens abroad and in the United States is an important strategic goal (37). Truly, HIV/AIDS is a very real threat to the health (physical, economic, political, etc.) of our world. And when the health and capabilities of nations are threatened, compromised, and even destroyed, international peacekeeping efforts and overall global security can become greatly compromised. A burgeoning realization that this scenario could occur in the developing world is encouraging government leaders, donor agencies, and other private and public organizations to respond with greater political and financial commitment to fight this HIV/AIDS pandemic.

Mobilization of Global Leadership and Resources

Global leadership has entered a new phase of cooperation to battle HIV/AIDS since the July 2000 conference in Durban. Many different organizations, national governments, international banking institutions, non-governmental organizations, private corporations, and pharmaceutical companies have joined in the global fight against the disease. The most notable result has been the creation of the Global Health Fund to fight HIV/AIDS, TB, and malaria under the leadership of United Nations Secretary-General Kofi Annan. First announced at the April 2001 African Summit on HIV, TB, and Other Related Infectious Diseases (ORID) in Abuja, Nigeria, its goal is to raise between $7 and $10 billion dollars a year to underwrite the health-care infrastructure and drugs needed to fight HIV and other infections.

Until now, public health threats that have attracted similar levels of international response have been natural disasters, such as famine, earthquakes, floods, and typhoons. The scale of global resource mobilization for HIV/AIDS may encourage similar efforts for other emerging infectious diseases, environmental problems, and bioterrorism. In fact, some level of global cooperation has occurred in several Western countries in response to bioterrorism-related anthrax cases occurring in the United States after the events of September 11, 2001. Specifically, this cooperation was demonstrated through Western countries and their collaboration in the global surveillance of anthrax and access to drugs.

Direct funding from the United States for international HIV/AIDS efforts continues to increase, with the fiscal year 2002 budget estimated at $760 million. This is up from $235 million in FY 2000 and $464.5 million in FY 2001 (42). Despite this positive trend, many experts argue that this amount is still not enough. Current HIV/AIDS prevention, care, and treatment programs in developing countries barely reach a small percentage of the population and those affected by the pandemic due to their meager funding base and financial resources, as well as small-scale programming. Increasingly, stakeholders are recognizing the urgent need for an expanded and comprehensive response to the global HIV/AIDS pandemic.

Health and Human Rights

The HIV epidemic has helped affirm the inextricable link between human rights and health. There is synergy between human rights and HIV/AIDS in that the extent to which individuals enjoy their human rights tends to define the degree to which they are vulnerable to HIV, and if infected with HIV, to which they are provided access to needed care, treatment, and support (43).

Instances of stigma and discrimination against people living with HIV, lack of confidentiality in HIV testing, inadequate access to prevention and care services, and denial of effective treatment in resource-poor settings have highlighted the importance of human rights in health. Often, the populations most severely affected by HIV are those who live on the fringes of society—those who are denied their human rights because of their behavior, gender, sexual orientation, ethnicity, race, or whatever social characteristic is stigmatized in a particular society (43). Stigmatized populations include sex workers, intravenous drug users, men who have sex with men, women, and youth. Other important factors that contribute to increased vulnerability of some populations include poverty, illiteracy, political instability, and war.

Human rights have long been recognized as important contributors to the attainment of health. However, the HIV/AIDS epidemic has increased the urgency for governments and societies to recognize, accept, and protect these rights. Especially important are the rights of individuals to consent to medical tests (e.g., HIV testing), respect for confidentiality for individuals' health information (e.g., HIV testing results), close involvement of patients in decision making for their care, and access to health resources.

Lack of national resources, inadequate health infrastructure, cost of drugs, patent rights, and protecting the investments of the pharmaceutical industry are no longer acceptable as reasons for denying treatment access to AIDS patients in poor countries. Advocacy groups, people living with HIV, and civil and political leaders have joined in the call to make HIV-related treatments available and affordable to poor countries. This has led to dramatic results: prices of anti-retroviral drugs have dropped dramatically, therapies have been offered at cost or free to developing countries, patent rights are being challenged and parallel importing is increasingly used, and resources are becoming available to provide treatment and care. Efforts to improve access to HIV/AIDS treatments will continue to evolve, raising the broader issue of affordable treatment for developing world citizens with other illnesses.

Patient Advocacy and Empowerment

Over the past twenty years, AIDS advocacy groups have made their mark on crucial policy issues, including human rights. People living with HIV in resource-rich countries demanded and obtained roles in diverse areas such as setting research priorities, designing policies relevant to AIDS, implementing the burgeoning HIV-oriented health services, and developing laws forbidding discrimination against persons infected with HIV. AIDS has also resulted in profound changes in patients' knowledge, rights, and involvement. Patients are now actively (rather than passively) involved in decision making in medical management.

As a result of this proactive approach in the domain of HIV/AIDS, other patient advocacy groups have been strengthened. For example, the mobilization of people living with breast and liver cancer, Parkinson's disease, and multiple sclerosis has led to successful advocacy for increased resources directed to these conditions (44).

Gender and HIV

The HIV/AIDS pandemic has underscored the issue of gender inequality. Women are more vulnerable to risks of HIV infection both biologically and economically (45,46). Biologically, the receptivity of the vagina, the greater area of susceptible tissue, and the mucosal micro trauma of sex make women more physiologically vulnerable to HIV. Socioeconomically, a woman's lack of access to education, her inability to generate income, and the gender sexual power imbalance create an even greater vulnerability to HIV infection. Finally, cultural traditions such as forced marriages, older men's preference for young women, and female genital mutilation all contribute to gender disempowerment (47).

Worldwide, prevailing views about masculinity encourage men to undertake risky sexual behaviors—multiple sex partners, alcohol consumption before intercourse, and sexual violence. Up to half of women worldwide report physical assault by an intimate partner (48). Young girls are at even greater risk of sexual coercion because they are perceived to be free of infection. Moreover, men control use of the main prevention tool to reduce risks of sexual transmission of HIV—the male condom (49). Finally, widespread poverty drives women into the sex industry where sexual trafficking and worker rotations promote continued exposure of new sex workers (and their clients) to HIV.

By highlighting the issue of gender inequity, the HIV epidemic has helped to mobilize the attention of world leaders to confront the underlying conditions, thus providing opportunities to improve women's health. International conferences in Cairo (1994) and Beijing (1995) have called for programs to improve women's access to education and employment. Activities to reduce sexual coercion and gender-based violence have also been initiated in a variety of country settings. Research on female-initiated microbicides to protect women against HIV has been gaining heightened advocacy by feminist organizations and additional funding by governments and foundations alike. Female controlled methods, such as microbicides, are intended to help reduce the gender power imbalance in negotiating safer sexual practices.

Heightened Awareness of Sexual Issues

Because HIV is predominantly transmitted by sexual behaviors, global programs aimed at preventing its spread have had to deal openly with the topic of sexual health. This has proven difficult for many cultures, given the highly private, morally charged, and frequently clandestine nature of sexual activities. Society's continued reluctance to openly confront sexual issues has perpetuated misperceptions about individual risk and promoted ignorance about the consequences of unprotected sexual behaviors (50). Debates at the June 2001 UNGASS over the appropriate wording to use with topics such as sexual orientation and condom use demonstrate that world leaders continue to experience discomfort when addressing sexual issues, even three decades into the course of the AIDS epidemic.

Nevertheless, as a direct result of the HIV epidemic, considerable progress has been made in increasing global awareness of sexual health issues (51). Many countries have undertaken national campaigns to communicate openly about sexual health and responsible sexual behaviors. Opinion leaders have been mobilized to address such sensitive issues as premarital sex, homosexuality, condom use, and sexual abuse. Sexuality education programs have been developed and professionals in a variety of settings—school, church, health facilities, and teen shelters—have been trained to raise, discuss, and counsel on sexuality topics. Even the mass media has been called on to provide prevention messages to counter the pervasive, sexually suggestive programs and advertisements that dominate their pages and airtime (52). While much more remains to be done globally, HIV has helped move sexual health from the "backwaters" of prurient gossip to the front lines of constructive public discussion and action.

For example, in 1999, the National Adolescent Sexual Health Initiative in South Africa launched a campaign called *loveLife* (53). This national, multimedia information and health service initiative uses brand-driven images to raise awareness of adolescent sexual health issues. Its main strategy is to help South Africans—particularly 12 to 17-year-olds—talk more openly about sex. *LoveLife* advocates a new lifestyle for young people based on informed choice, shared responsibility, and positive sexuality (53).

The initial evaluation of the *loveLife* awareness campaign showed that the positive outcomes of the branding messages (e.g., reducing unsafe sex) markedly outweighed the negative outcomes (e.g., increased sexual experimentation). However, the process evaluations indicated that the campaign was less successful in sparking a national discourse about sexuality than it was in stimulating thought about the issues raised by the campaign (53).

Impact on Global Public Health Structure and Technology

In general, the building of a health infrastructure in resource-poor settings has been considered beyond the realm of feasibility, even for major resource donors. However, this hesitancy has been overcome by heightened interest in the HIV epidemic, coupled with the breadth of resource commitments among public and private funders.

Although it in no way compensates for the huge toll on human capital described earlier, investments in HIV prevention and care have served an important capacity-building function in resource-poor settings. The multifaceted global response to HIV has involved a variety of public health and clinical approaches, each implemented to varying degrees in multiple countries, depending on such factors as political will, magnitude of the epidemic, and the previous health infrastructure (54,55). HIV-related activities such as public education, other community prevention efforts, programs to improve nutritional status, and the provision of health services—including palliative care, treatment of opportunistic infections, and, eventually, antiretrovirals—have and will contribute to broadly increasing global health capacity (54,55).

Moreover, the fruits of two decades of research, largely conducted in resource-rich settings, can now be impressively marshaled for global public health. Attempts to deliver both HIV vaccines and treatments will provide a springboard for investment in organizational structures and accessible technology for the developing world.

Conclusion

The HIV/AIDS epidemic continues its global spread. To successfully control further worldwide transmission of this virus, we need to apply, on a much larger scale, the lessons learned from the past two decades. Strategies that have proven effective in HIV prevention, care, support, and treatment must be replicated in a variety of global settings to create an optimal "herd effect" in slowing HIV spread. The earlier in the stage of HIV infection we are able to intervene, the more targeted and effective our prevention approaches can be (56).

Ironically, precisely because of its unparalleled devastation, the HIV/AIDS epidemic has helped to positively change the future of global public health on multiple fronts: by marshalling the world's attention to the health status of resource-poor countries, by demonstrating the inextricable link between human rights and human health, by raising the profile of sexual health within global preventive medicine, by heightening the need for gender empowerment in negotiating safer behaviors, thus ensuring improved health for women, and by "raising the bar" for the level of resources necessary to support health infrastructures to prevent and treat HIV and its associated diseases.

References

1. Annan, K: Presentation at the Global Health Council's Annual Meeting's Banquet, Washington, DC, June 1, 2001.
2. UNAIDS Press Release: *Momentum Builds for UN Special Session on HIV/AIDS: Secretary-General's Call for Action Sets Stage for Negotiations This Week.* New York, May 21, 2001.
3. UNAIDS: *AIDS Epidemic Update, December 2001 and UNAIDS Report on the Global HIV/AIDS Epidemic: New HIV Estimates.* New York, December 2000.
4. URL: www.aids.about.com, Adler M: ABC of AIDS: Development of the epidemic; *Br Med J* 322: 1226–1229, 2001.
5. Population Reference Bureau (PRB): *2000 World Population Data Sheet: Demographic Data and Estimates for the Countries and Regions of the World.* PRB, Washington, DC, 2000.
6. Delay P, Stanecki K, and G Ernberg: Introduction. In Lamptey PR and Gayle HD (eds.): *HIV/AIDS Prevention and Care in Resource-Constrained Settings: A Handbook for the Design and Management of Programs.* Arlington, VA: Family Health International AIDS Institute, 2001, pp. VII–XXV.
7. Stanecki K: US Census Bureau, International Data Base and unpublished tables, 2000.
8. Alban A and Guinness L: *Socio-Economic Impact of HIV/AIDS in Africa,* ADF/UNAIDS 2000 presentation in PowerPoint. December 3–7, 2000 Addis Ababa, Ethiopia.
9. UNICEF: Survey from CAR, 1999 in *Socio-Economic Impact of HIV/AIDS in Africa* ADF/UNAIDS 2000 presentation in PowerPoint. December3–7, 2000. Addis Ababa, Ethiopia.
10. Bateman C: Can KwaZulu-Natal hospitals cope with the HIV/AIDS human tide? *S Afr Med J* 91(5): 364–368, 2001.
11. Stover J: *The Impact of HIV/AIDS on Population Growth in Africa.* Futures Group International, Washington, DC, 1993.
12. Colvin M et al.: Prevalence of HIV and HIV-related diseases in the adult medical wards of a tertiary hospital in Durban, South Africa. *Int J STD AIDS* 12(6): 386–389, 2001.

13. Schneider P, et al.: Paper presented at International AIDS Economics Network symposium, 2000 from *Socio-Economic Impact of HIV/AIDS in Africa*, ADF/UNAIDS 2000 presentation in PowerPoint.

14. Kwaramba P: Presentation from *Socio-Economic Impact of HIV/AIDS in Africa*, ADF/UNAIDS 2000 presentation in PowerPoint. 3–7 December 2000, Addis Ababa, Ethiopia.

15. Family Health International: *Economic Impact of AIDS*. FHI, Arlington, VA, 1999.

16. Turner M: Zimbabwe losing ground against disease.*Financial Times*, July 2, 2001.

17. Jones C: Presentation from *Socio-economic Impact of HIV/AIDS in Africa* ADF/UNAIDS 2000 presentation in PowerPoint.

18. WHO/WPRO: 100 percent condom use programme in entertainment establishments, Annex 1—Thailand Case Study. World Health Organization 2000 Geneva.

19. Wasserheit JN: Epidemiological synergy: interrelationships between human immunodeficiency virus infection and other sexually transmitted diseases. *Sex Transm Dis* 19: 61–77, 1992.

20. Cates W Jr: The "other STIs": Do they matter? *JAMA* 259: 3606–3608, 1988.

21. Grosskurth H, Mosha F, Todd J, et al.: Impact of improved treatment of sexually transmitted diseases on HIV infection in rural Tanzania: randomized controlled trial. *Lancet* 346: 530–536, 1995.

22. Gilson L, Mkanje R, Grosskurth H, et al.: Cost-effectiveness of improved treatment services for sexually transmitted diseases in preventing HIV-1 infection in Mwanza Region, Tanzania. *Lancet* 350: 1805–1809, 1997.

23. Wawer MJ, Sewankambo NK, Serwadda D, et al.: Control of sexually transmitted diseases for AIDS prevention in Uganda: a randomized community trial. *Lancet* 353: 525–535, 1999.

24. Steen R, Vulsteke B, De Coito T, et al.: Evidence of declining STD prevalence in a South Afrian mining community followng core-group intervention. *Sex Transm Dis* 27: 1–8, 2000.

25. Hayes R, Wawer M, Gray R, et al.: Randomized trials of STI treatment for HIV prevention: Report of an international workshop. *Genitourin Med* 73: 432–443, 1997.

26. Grosskurth H, Gray R, Hayes R, Mabey D, and Wawer M: Control of sexually transmitted diseases for HIV-1 prevention: understanding the implications of the Mwanza and Rakai trials. *Lancet* 355: WA8–WA14, 2000.

27. Boily MC, Lowndes CM, and Alary M: Complimentary hypothesis concerning the community sexually transmitted mass treatment puzzle in Rakai, Uganda. *AIDS* 14: 2583–2592, 2000.

28. Cohen MS, Hoffman IF, Royce RA, et al.: Reduction of concentration of HIV-1 in semen after treatment of urethritis: implications for prvention of sexual transmission of HIV-1. *Lancet* 349: 1868–1873, 1997.

29. Quinn TC, Wawer MJ, Sewankambo NK, et al.: Viral load and heterosexual transmission of human immune deficiency virus type 1. *N Engl J Med* 342: 921–929, 2000.

30. Coates T, et al.: The Voluntary HIV-1 Counseling and Testing Efficacy Study Group. Efficacy of voluntary HIV-1 counseling and testing in individuals and couples in Kenya, Tanzania and Trinidad: a randomized trial. *Lancet* 356: 103–112, 2000.

31. Mofenson L and McIntyre J: Advances and research direction in the prevention of mother-to-child HIV-1 transmission. *Lancet* 355: WA27–WA34, 2000.

32. De Cock KM, Fowler MG, Mercier E, de Vincenzi I, Saba J, Hoff E, Alnwick DJ, Rogers M, and Shaffer N: Prevention of mother-to-child HIV transmission in resource-poor countries: translating research into policy and practice. *JAMA* 283: 1175–1182, 2000.

33. Guay LA, Musoke P, Fleming T, et al.: Intrapartum and neonatal single-dose nevi-rapine compared with zidovudine for prevention of mother-to-child transmission of HIV-1 in Kampala, Uganda: HIVNET 012 randomised trial. *Lancet* 354: 795–802, 1999.

34. Soderlund N, Zwi K, Kinghorn A, and Gray G: Prevention of vertical transmission of HIV: analysis of cost effectiveness of options available in South Africa. *Br Med J* 318: 1650–1656, 1999.

35. Miotti PG, Taha TET, Kumwenda NI, et al.: HIV transmission through breastfeeding: a study in Malawi. *JAMA* 282: 744–749, 1999.

36. Nduati R, John G, Mbori-Ngacha D, et al.: Effect of breastfeeding and formula feed-ing on transmission of HIV-1: a randomized clinical trial. *JAMA* 283: 1167–1174, 2000.

37. National Intelligence Council: *The Global Infectious Disease Threat and Its Impli-cations for the United States.* CIA Washington, DC, 2000.

38. World Health Organization, World Health Day 1997: Press Release WHO/28 "Emerg-ing Infectious Diseases, Global Alert–Global Response," April 4, 1997.

39. U.S. State Department: CISET Task Force on Emerging and Infectious Diseases. www.state.gov /www/global/oes/health/task_force/index.html#ciset.

40. International Crises Group: *HIV/AIDS as a Security Issue.* Washington DC, Interna-tional Crises Group, 2001.

41. Lobe J: *HEALTH: The Spread of AIDS Seen as Security Threat.* Inter Press Service. June 20, 2001.

42. San Francisco AIDS Foundation: *HIV Advocacy Network Information Alert: 106th Congress Comes to a Close: HIV Programs Receive Significant Funding Increases.* www.saf.org accessed June 2001.

43. Gruskin S and Tarantola D: HIV/AIDS, health and human rights. In Lamptey PR and Gayle HD (eds.): *HIV/AIDS Prevention and Care in Resource-Constrained Settings: A Handbook for the Design and Management of Programs.* Family Health Interna-tional AIDS Institute, Arlington, VA, 2001.

44. Arno PS and KL Feiden: *Against the Odds: The Story of AIDS Drug Development, Politics, and Profits.* New York: HarperCollins, 1992.

45. UNAIDS: *Gender and HIV/AIDS: Taking Stock of Research and Programmes.* Geneva, March 1999.

46. A gendered edpidemic: women and the risks and burdens of HIV. *JAMWA* 56: 90–91.

47. Gomez CA and Marin BV: Gender, culture, and power: barriers to HIV-prevention strategies for women. *J Sex Res* 33(4): 355–362, 1996.

48. Heise L, Ellsberg M, and Gottemoeller M: *Ending Violence against Women* (Popula-tion Reports, Series L, No. 11). Johns Hopkins University School of Public Health, Population Information Program, Baltimore, 1999.

49. NIAID: *Workshop Summary: Scientific Evidence on Condom Effectiveness for Sexu-ally Transmitted Disease (STD) Prevention.* June 12–13, Hyatt Dulles Airport, Hern-don, VA Report prepared July 2001.

50. Institute of Medicine: No time to lose: getting more from HIV prevention. In Ruiz MS, et al.: (eds.): National Academy Press, Washington, DC, 2000, pp. 100.

51. Satcher DA: *The Surgeon General's Call to Action to Promote Sexual Health and Re-sponsible Sexual Behavior.* Washington, DC, Office of the U.S. Surgeon General, 2001.

52. Huston AC, Wartella E, and Donnerstein E: *Measuring the Effects of Sexual Content in the Media: A Report to the Kaiser Family Foundation.* Kaiser Family Foundation, Menlo Park, 1998.

53. Stadler J: *loveLife: The First Year.* Reproductive Health Research Unit, Johannesburg, 2001.

54. Folkers GK and Fauci AS: The AIDS research model: implications for other infectious diseases of global health importance. *JAMA* 286: 458–461, 2001.

55. Satcher D: Global HIV/AIDS revisited. *JAMA* 286: 25–35, 2001.

56. Garnett GP and Anderson RM: Strategies for limited the spread of HIV in developing countries: conclusions based on studies of the transmission dynamics of the virus. *J Acquir Immune Defic Syndr Hum Retrovirol* 9: 500–513, 1995.

Epilogue

The HIV Epidemic's Effect on the Training and Practice of Future Public Health Professionals

JAMES W. CURRAN

The human immunodeficiency virus (HIV) epidemic poses a great threat to public health. The biologic and social complexity of HIV challenges our skills and encourages us to direct scientific efforts and use new approaches to prevent HIV, care for those affected, and slow the epidemic. The explosive spread of HIV throughout the world provides many lessons and teaches public health professionals humility, a clear sense of urgency, and the need for a global perspective.

HIV as a New Disease

The first cases of what is now termed acquired immunodeficiency syndrome (AIDS) were recognized in 1981 (1). Subsequently, cases of AIDS were recognized throughout the world, and epidemics of serious illness and death followed. Within three years of the syndrome's recognition, the virus responsible for AIDS, human immunodeficiency virus (HIV), was discovered. This led to a clearer understanding of the natural history of the infection and an appreciation of the extent of the epidemic.

Indeed, in 1981 the HIV epidemic was "new"—previously unrecognized as a human infection, except for rare cases detected prior to the 1970s. The spread of this virus throughout the world has been both insidious and explosive, aided by the fact that infection typically precedes serious clinical symptoms and detection by many years. Furthermore, HIV infection invariably persists in the human host, leading to large-scale global endemicity—a human reservoir of infection numbering in the tens of millions. And HIV's attack on the immune system renders those infected susceptible to many other infections, thus facilitating the spread of tuberculosis and other infections.

The HIV/AIDS epidemic awakened the world to the reality and implications of resurgent infectious disease. This awareness has been heightened by outbreaks of Ebola virus, microbial contamination of food, and anthrax spread by terrorists. The AIDS epidemic, along with these other very real threats, serve as a "call to action" for a generation of young public health professionals and students. The complex challenge of HIV/AIDS brings out the best in those who have a mission to prevent and care for those affected by this virus.

The HIV Epidemic Is Complex

Nothing about AIDS is simple. HIV, as an RNA retrovirus, integrates into the DNA of multiple human cell types and persists for the life of the host. Its capacity to change (viral heterogeneity) is well known; the pathogenesis of disease is incompletely understood; and for most, disease progression remains inexorable in the absence of therapy. HIV is present in blood and body fluids such as semen and vaginal secretions, meaning that the vast majority of infections are transmitted through intimate and private human behaviors—sexual intercourse; bearing, delivering, and breast feeding an infant; or injecting drugs with contaminated equipment. Most HIV infections in the world are transmitted and acquired without specific knowledge of the risks involved, since the majority of persons infected with HIV are initially unaware of their infection status.

Along with its biologic variability, stigma and other social variables greatly add to the complexity of the epidemic. A major lesson from the HIV epidemic is that the environment greatly influences the spread of infection. In any society, the linking of a life-threatening infection to sexual intercourse will result in a high level of stigma and subsequent discrimination against those infected. But poverty and social disorder exacerbate the situation by combining with personal and societal denial and discrimination to inhibit HIV awareness and prevention efforts.

The Road Map for Public Health

Countless thousands of students, volunteers, and workers throughout the world have responded to the challenge of the HIV epidemic and strengthened the public health response. How best can these workers prepare for this challenge, and will the public health response be adequate?

Public health has been defined as "what we, as a society, do collectively to assure the conditions in which people can be healthy" (2). Public health, then, is not synonymous with public (or governmental) medicine but, rather, involves multiple disciplines and broader input. Accomplishing the public health mission requires contributions from private individuals and organizations, as well as public agencies. It is government's responsibility, however, to assure the accomplishment of the mission by either coordinating or otherwise providing the necessary elements of public health programs. The Institute of Medicine (IOM) Committee on the Future of Public Health described government's core public health functions as assessment, policy, development, and assurance (2).

The assessment role for HIV prevention and care begins with surveillance of HIV/AIDS and high-risk behaviors (Chapter 2), as well as community needs (Chapter 3), and should include detailed knowledge of available prevention and care programs known to be efficient, effective, and acceptable. Development of effective HIV policies begins with an adequate science base for determining effective prevention and treatment priorities (Chapters 4 and 8). Effective policy formulation requires developing consensus (Chapter 3) and crafting and evaluating laws and regulations (Chapters 5, 6, and 7). Fulfilling the core function of assurance remains the biggest challenge for public health. This is especially apparent for prevention of HIV and care for persons with HIV throughout the world (Chapter 9). Even in the United States, costly care is often not available for those infected with HIV, and programs to prevent HIV infection and injecting drug use are chronically underfunded. The stigma due to HIV infection and the relative poverty of many of those at highest risk make the assurance role all the more difficult (as Chapter 6 indicates).

Public health has the tools to prevent HIV infection and care for HIV disease. Effective programs begin with science. The science base for HIV prevention and care has dramatically improved, although a cure remains elusive and treatment failures and costs of care are major concerns. In addition to curative therapy, the development and testing of a safe and effective HIV vaccine is our highest research priority. Such a discovery is critical for the long-term success of global prevention efforts. HIV prevention research has provided us with effective methods to reduce HIV transmission in most settings, but few such efforts have been "scaled up" and truly evaluated at larger geographic levels, and funding for HIV prevention throughout the world remains grossly inadequate.

The skills taught to students of public health are valuable to the HIV workforce, and the mix of skills, likewise, has been informed by the HIV epidemic. Skills in epidemiology and biostatistics are needed to assess this and future epidemics, as well as to evaluate programmatic needs and activities. Health education, counseling, and health communication courses will provide public health workers the skills needed to educate the public and populations at risk. Courses in health policy and management provide skills to manage programs and evaluate programmatic activities and to understand and craft effective policies. The HIV epidemic has reinforced for many of us in public health the crucial role that those in the community play in designing and advocating for effective programs for their own communities. In particular, the leadership provided by HIV-infected persons has often been successful in bridging gaps between government and community.

Leadership and the Future

The HIV epidemic continues to expand throughout the world, and a global perspective is needed to assess the problem and develop strategies for prevention and control. Commitment to research for an effective vaccine and curative therapy remains crucial. Review of the short history of the HIV epidemic reveals many successes in HIV prevention and care. Progress has been based on science, but successful implementation relies on public health workers and community members working together. The future challenges will also require the same commitment, collaborations, and leadership. As the late Jonathan Mann noted:

Our responsibility is historic. For when the history of AIDS and the global response is written, our most precious contribution may well be that at a time of plague, we did not flee, we did not hide, we did not separate ourselves. (3)

References

1. Centers for Disease Control: *Pneumocystis pneumonia*—Los Angeles. *Morb Mortal Wkly Rep* 30: 250–252, 1981.
2. *The Future of Public Health*, National Academy Press, Washington, DC, 1988, pp. 1–18. Institute of Medicine, Committee for the Study of the Future of Public Health.
3. Mann JM: Presentation at the Thirteenth International Conference on AIDS, Geneva, Switzerland, June 30, 1998.

Index